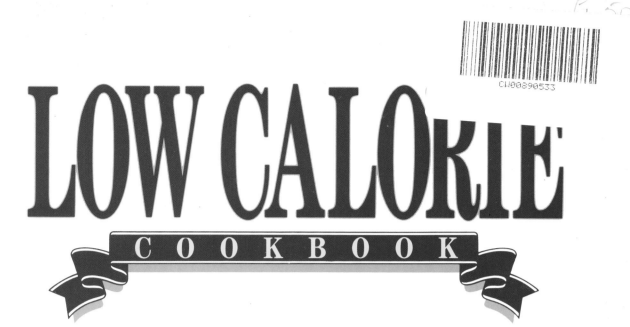

LOW CALORIE COOKBOOK

If you're one of the lucky few who don't have to watch your waistline or worry about what you eat – the other 99 per cent of us ordinary mortals envy you! But, even you probably have to plan meals for your family. So we're all in the same calorie-conscious boat.

Here, we have created a book full of quick and easy recipes that will help you keep your weight under control in the most delicious way.

Every recipe has been calorie/kilojoule counted and designed to give you maximum flavour and satisfaction, while at the same time helping you lose weight.

If you have a cholesterol problem, this book will work very well for you, too. We suggest you substitute margarine or oil for butter, if used.

In a sensible weight reduction regime, dietary fibre plays a very important part. And, of course, before going on any diet you should always check with your doctor first.

For more handy information about dieting please turn to page 48.

Editor Philip Gore **Design** Craig Osment **Art Director** Stephen Joseph **Cookery Editor** Loukie Werle **Food Stylist** Wendy Berecry **Food for Photography** Belinda Clayton **Photography** Warren Webb **Research Assistant** Penelope Peel **Editorial Production** Margaret Gore & Associates **Typesetting** APT Pty Ltd **Printed** in Japan by Dai Nippon, Tokyo **Published** by Century Magazines Pty Ltd, 216-224 Commonwealth Street, Surry Hills, NSW 2010, Australia. **UK Distribution** T.B. Clarke (UK) Distributors, Beckett House, 14 Billing Road, Northampton NN1 5AW. Tel: (0604) 23 0941. Fax: (0604) 23 0942. **Australian Distribution** (Supermarkets) Select Magazines Pty Ltd, Suite 402, 7 Merriwa Street, Gordon, NSW 2072. (Newsagents) NDD 150 Bourke Road, Alexandria, NSW 2015. ©**Century Magazines Pty Ltd** *Recommended retail price. **Photography Credits** We gratefully acknowledge **David Jones** Bondi Junction; **Barbara's House and Garden** Birkenhead Point; **Australia East India Company** Bondi Junction; **Villa Italiana** Mosman; **Accoutrement** Mosman; **Fred Pazotti** Woollahra; **Made Where** Double Bay; **The Design Store** Spit Junction; **Opus** Paddington; **Hale Imports** Brookvale; **Casa Shopping** Darlinghurst; **Country Floors** Woollahra.

SLIMMING SOUPS

Here's a delicious selection of summer and winter soups that are high in flavour and low in kilojoules.

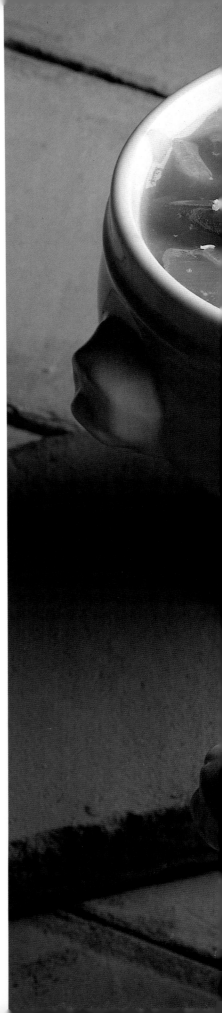

Minestrone with Pesto

628 kilojoules/150 calories per serving

PESTO

2 cups fresh basil leaves

6 large cloves garlic, crushed

1 tblspn olive oil

MINESTRONE

1 tblspn light butter

½ onion, peeled and chopped

1 leek, washed and sliced

1 carrot, peeled and sliced

1 celery stalk, cut into slices

1 clove garlic, crushed

2 tomatoes, chopped

4 cabbage leaves, chopped

1 cup sliced green beans

6 cups chicken stock

¼ cup grated pecorino cheese

1 To make pesto: Place basil leaves, garlic cloves and oil in a blender and process until mixture is very finely chopped. Pour mixture into an ice cube tray and freeze until ready to use.

2 To make the minestrone: Melt the butter in a large frying pan over a medium heat. Add the onion, leek, carrot, celery, garlic, tomatoes, cabbage and beans, cook for 2 minutes stirring constantly. Add the stock and bring to the boil. Lower the heat and simmer, uncovered, for 20 minutes.

3 Serve soup in large heated soup bowls, place a pesto cube in each bowl and sprinkle with the cheese.

Serves 6

Borscht

502 kilojoules/120 calories per serving

1 potato, peeled and cut into 1cm (½in) cubes

8 beets, peeled and cut into 1cm (½in) cubes

10 cups chicken stock

30g (1oz) unsalted butter

2 onions, finely chopped

2 carrots, peeled and cut into 0.5cm (¼in) cubes

2 cups finely chopped white cabbage

2 large tomatoes, peeled, seeded and finely chopped

8 tblspn plain low fat yoghurt

2 tblspn chopped fresh dill

1 Simmer potatoes and beets in chicken stock for 10-12 minutes, or until tender. Strain, reserving both stock and vegetables.

2 Melt butter in a saucepan, add onion, saute until translucent. Add carrots, cabbage, tomatoes and reserved stock. Simmer, covered, for 20 minutes. Add potatoes and beets and cook until heated through.

3 Serve hot in heated individual bowls, with 1 tablespoon yoghurt and a sprinkling of fresh dill in each bowl.

Serves 8

Minestrone with Pesto

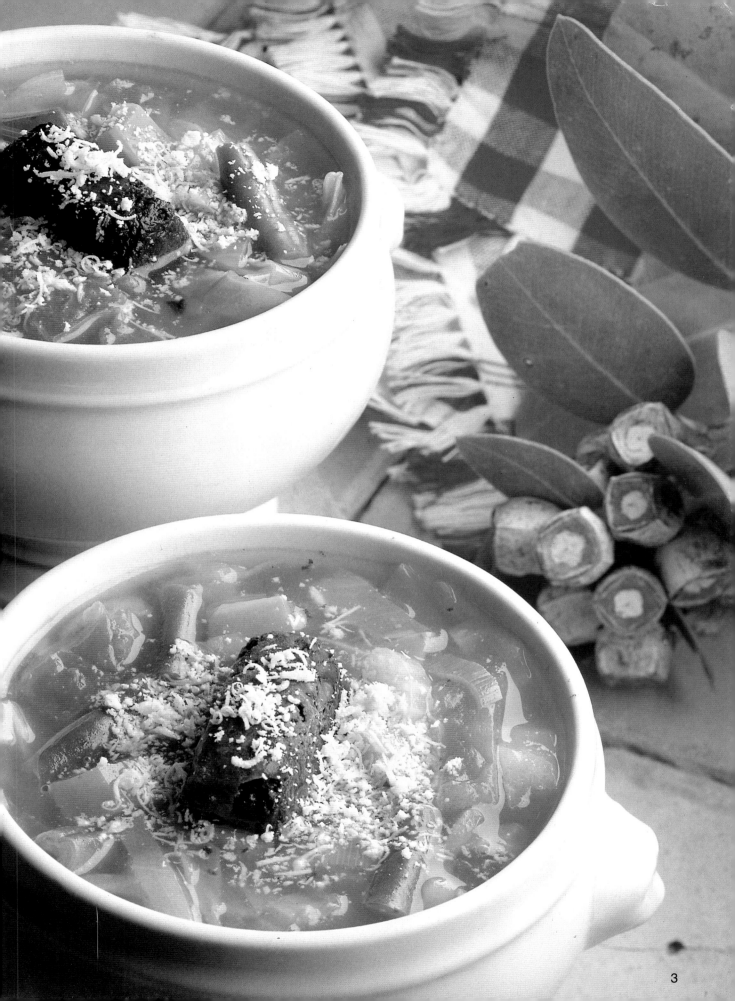

Cauliflower and Coriander Soup

183 kilojoules/45 calories per serving

1 tblspn lite margarine

1 onion, peeled and finely chopped

2 cups cauliflowerets, cut into small pieces

1 tblspn chopped fresh coriander

2 bay leaves

4 cups chicken stock

½ cup skim milk

¼ tspn black cracked pepper

1 Melt the margarine in a large saucepan over a moderate heat. Add the onion and cook for 2 minutes, stir in the cauliflower, coriander and bay leaves, cook for a further 5 minutes, stirring constantly.

2 Add the stock, milk and pepper and bring to the boil. Reduce heat and simmer uncovered for 20 minutes.

3 Cool mixture slightly and puree in a food processor or blender until smooth.

4 Reheat soup before serving and garnish with fresh coriander.

Serves 4

Vegetable Soup

84 kilojoules/20 calories per serving

8 cups vegetable stock (recipe follows)

100g (3½oz) carrots, thinly sliced

100g (3½oz) French beans, finely chopped

60g (2oz) cauliflowerets, cut into small pieces

60g (2oz) peas

60g (2oz) broccoli flowerets, cut into small pieces

salt

pepper

parsley for garnish

1 Bring stock to a boil. Add carrots, beans, cauliflower and peas. Simmer 5 minutes.

2 Add broccoli and cook 2-3 minutes or until tender.

3 Season to taste with salt and freshly ground pepper. Serve hot, garnished with parsley.

Serves 8

Vegetable Stock

negligible kilojoules/calories

10 cups water

3 onions, roughly chopped

4 celery stalks, chopped

4 carrots, peeled and sliced

2 zucchini (courgette), rinsed and sliced

4 tomatoes, seeded and chopped

2 cloves garlic

1 bay leaf

1 bouquet garni

8 black peppercorns

1 Place all ingredients into a large saucepan. Bring to a boil. Reduce heat to a simmer, cook uncovered for 10 minutes. Strain and cool.

Makes about 10 cups

Scallop, Tomato and Fennel Soup

502 kilojoules/120 calories per serving

4 tblspn olive oil

2 large onions, thinly sliced

3 small fennel bulbs, thinly sliced, reserve feathery leaves for garnish

3 cloves garlic, thinly sliced

1kg (2lb) ripe tomatoes, peeled, chopped

⅛ tspn cayenne pepper

salt

8 cups degreased fish stock (recipe follows)

40 scallops

1 Heat oil in a saucepan, add onion, fennel and garlic. Cook over low heat for 10 minutes, stirring occasionally.

2 Stir in tomatoes and cayenne pepper, season to taste with salt. Add fish stock and bring to a boil. Reduce heat and simmer 35-40 minutes or until fennel is tender.

3 Allow to cool slightly, puree in a blender or processor and return to saucepan. Bring to a simmer, add scallops and cook until heated through, about 3 minutes. Serve hot, garnished with fennel leaves.

Serves 8

Fish Stock

21 kilojoules/5 calories per serving

500g (1lb) fish bones from white fleshed fish

1 onion, sliced

1 stalk celery, sliced

6 stalks parsley

¼ cup chopped mushrooms

2 cups white wine

12 cups water

1 Rinse fish bones under cold running water, place in a large saucepan with remaining ingredients and bring to a boil.

2 Reduce heat, simmer, uncovered, for 25 minutes. Strain through a fine sieve. Allow to cool, cover, refrigerate to allow any fat to rise to surface. Remove fat.

Makes about 14 cups

Gazpacho

357 kilojoules/85 calories per serving

½ onion, roughly chopped

½ cucumber, peeled and seeded

½ green capsicum (pepper), seeded and roughly chopped

1 clove garlic, crushed

1 tblspn chopped coriander

1½ cups Italian peeled tomatoes

1 cup tomato puree

1 tblspn red wine vinegar

1 tspn lemon juice

¼ tspn Tabasco sauce

1 stick celery, chopped, for garnish

1 Place all ingredients, except celery, in a blender or food processor and blend for 30 seconds.

2 Chill soup before serving and garnish with chopped celery.

Serves 4

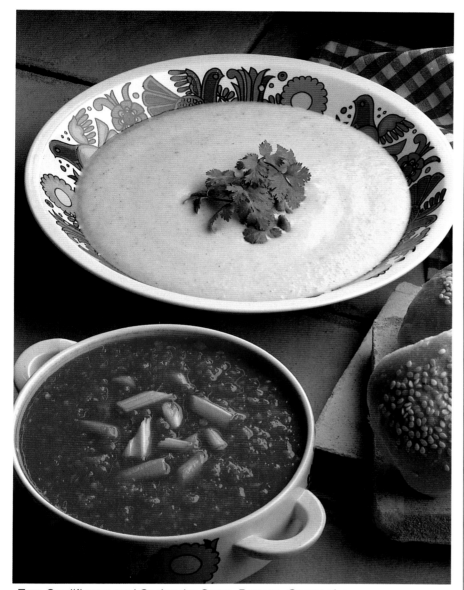

Top: Cauliflower and Coriander Soup. Bottom: Gazpacho

Chinese-style Bouillon

837 kilojoules/200 calories per serving

315g (10oz) lean, boneless beef

4 tblspn tamari (see note 1)

3 tspn plain flour

salt

pepper

1 tblspn mustard seed oil (see note 2)

6 cups degreased hot beef stock

3 small carrots, julienned

185g (6oz) bamboo shoots, drained, rinsed and julienned

12 medium mushrooms, sliced

6-8 shitake mushrooms, sliced

4 cups bean sprouts

45g (1½oz) transparent noodles, cut into short lengths

10 spinach leaves, finely chopped

250g (½lb) firm tofu, cut into thin strips

1 tblspn dry sherry

1 Cut beef into paper-thin strips. Marinate in combined tamari and flour, seasoned to taste with salt and freshly ground pepper, for 10 minutes.

2 Heat oil in a heavy pan, add beef strips with marinade, saute until browned on all sides. Add heated stock, carrots and bamboo shoots. Simmer 5 minutes.

3 Stir in mushrooms, sprouts and noodles, cook 5 minutes. Add spinach and tofu, heat through. Add sherry, adjust seasoning. Serve hot.

Note 1: Tamari is like soy sauce, but stronger flavoured. It is available in health food shops.

Note 2: Mustard Seed Oil is a highly polyunsaturated oil, available at selected food halls and some speciality food shops.

Serves 6

Chilled Indian Cucumber Soup

398 kilojoules/95 calories per serving

1 bunch fresh coriander

2 onions, roughly chopped

4 cucumbers, peeled, seeded and sliced

2½ cups plain low fat yoghurt

1 tspn curry powder

4 drops Tabasco sauce

salt

pepper

2 cups degreased chicken stock

⅓ cup plain low fat yoghurt for garnish

coriander leaves for garnish

1 Wash coriander thoroughly. Chop leaves and stalks in a processor. Add onions and cucumber, process until finely chopped.

2 In a bowl combine yoghurt with curry powder and Tabasco, season to taste with salt and freshly ground pepper.

3 Whisk chicken stock and cucumber mixture into yoghurt. Cover and refrigerate at least 2 hours.

4 Serve in chilled bowls and garnish with a dollop of yoghurt and fresh coriander leaves.

Serves 8

Vichyssoise

293 kilojoules/70 calories per serving

1 tspn lite margarine

3 leeks, sliced

1 onion, peeled and sliced

2 large potatoes, peeled and chopped

4 cups degreased chicken stock

½ cup non-fat skim milk

1 tblspn chopped fresh chives

1 Melt the margarine in a large saucepan over a medium heat. Add the leeks, onion and potatoes and cook for 3 minutes, stirring constantly.

2 Pour in the stock and bring to the boil, reduce heat and simmer, covered, for 30 minutes.

3 Place mixture and skim milk into a food processor or blender and process until smooth. Refrigerate for 3 hours and serve in chilled bowls, garnished with chives.

Serves 4

Curried Carrot and Chive Soup

293 kilojoules/70 calories per serving

1 tblspn butter

2 large onions, chopped

8 carrots, peeled and chopped

6 stalks parsley, chopped

1 clove garlic, sliced

3 tblspn curry powder (more if desired)

10 cups degreased chicken stock

pepper

1 bunch chives, chopped

1 Melt butter in a large heavy-based saucepan. Add onion, carrots, parsley stalks and garlic. Sweat over low heat for 4-5 minutes, being careful not to brown vegetables.

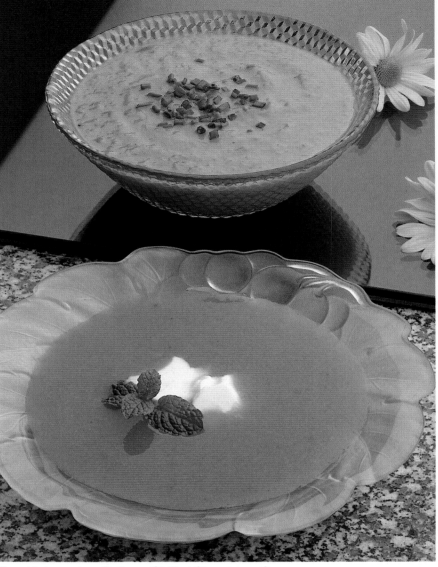

Top: Vichyssoise. Bottom: Chilled Strawberry Soup

2 Stir in curry powder and cook, stirring constantly, for 2-3 minutes. Make sure curry does not burn.

3 Add stock, bring to a boil. Reduce heat to a simmer and cook for 30 minutes or until vegetables are tender. Puree in a blender or processor.

4 Return soup to saucepan, season to taste with freshly ground pepper, reheat. Serve hot, sprinkled with chopped chives.

Serves 8

Chilled Strawberry Soup

293 kilojoules/70 calories per serving

2 cups strawberries, hulled and washed

½ cup apple juice

½ cup orange juice

¼ cup natural skim milk yoghurt

mint for garnish

1 Place the strawberries, apple juice and orange juice into a blender or food processor, puree until smooth.

2 Pour mixture into chilled glasses or bowls, swirl a teaspoon of yoghurt on the top and garnish with fresh mint if desired.

Serves 6

Iced Watercress and Lemon Soup

167 kilojoules/40 calories per serving

2 bunches watercress, stalks removed and chopped

1 onion, finely chopped

2 cups degreased chicken stock

1 cup skim milk

2 tspn grated lemon rind

¼ tspn black pepper

½ cup natural yoghurt

1 Wash the watercress and place in a large saucepan (reserve a few sprigs for garnish) with the onion, stock, milk, lemon rind and pepper.

2 Simmer gently for 25 minutes, then puree mixture in a blender or processor until smooth.

3 Stir in the yoghurt and chill. Serve soup chilled and garnish with a sprig of watercress.

Serves 6

Mushroom and Barley Soup

335 kilojoules/80 calories per serving

500g (1lb) fresh button mushrooms, sliced

1 small tomato, quartered

2 medium carrots, peeled and chopped

1 onion, chopped

2 celery stalks, chopped

½ tspn salt

4 parsley sprigs, chopped

½ cup barley

fresh chopped parsley, to garnish

1 In a large saucepan combine the mushrooms, tomato, carrots, onion, celery, salt, parsley, barley and 6 cups of water.

2 Bring to the boil, reduce heat and simmer covered for 1 hour. Serve hot and garnish with fresh parsley.

Serves 4

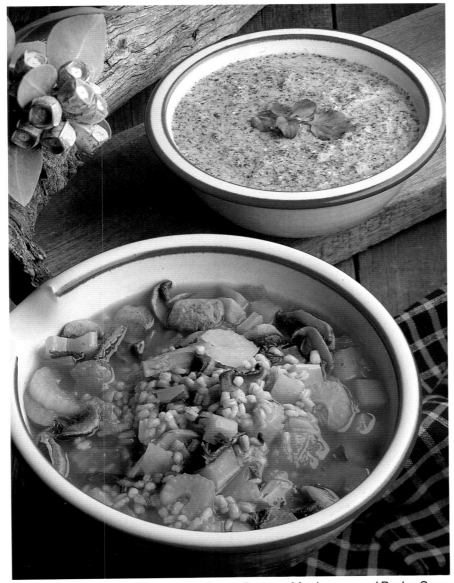

Top: Iced Watercress and Lemon Soup. Bottom: Mushroom and Barley Soup

Cheese and Parsnip Soup

712 kilojoules/170 calories per serving

1 tspn unsalted butter

2 large onions, peeled and chopped

2 tspn caraway seeds

185g (6oz) fennel, chopped

1 large potato, scrubbed and chopped

2 stalks celery, chopped

500g (1lb) parsnips, peeled and sliced

6 cups vegetable stock (see page 4)

60g (2oz) low fat Cheddar cheese, grated

salt

pepper

caraway seeds for garnish

1 Heat butter in a heavy saucepan, add onion and caraway seeds, cook until onion is soft and golden. Add fennel, potato, celery and parsnip, sweat vegetables for 3-4 minutes. Do not brown.

2 Add stock to vegetables. Bring to a boil, cover and simmer 20-25 minutes, or until vegetables are tender. Cool, puree in a blender or processor until smooth.

3 Return mixture to saucepan, bring to a boil. Add cheese, season to taste with salt and freshly ground pepper. Simmer until cheese melts. Serve hot, garnished with caraway seeds.

Serves 8

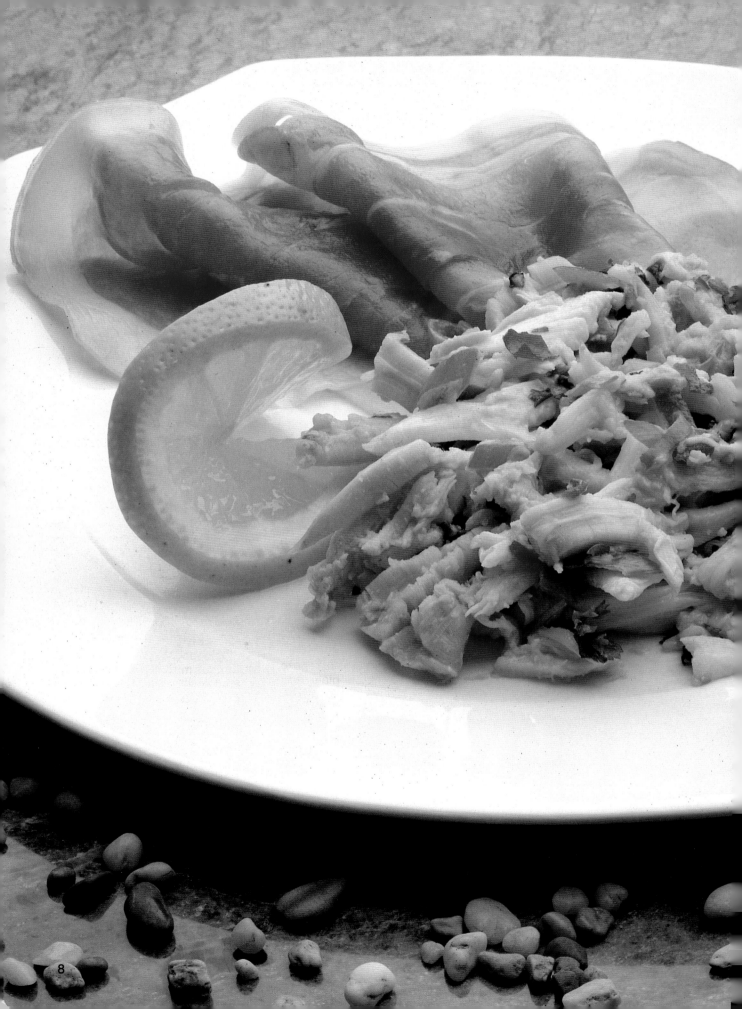

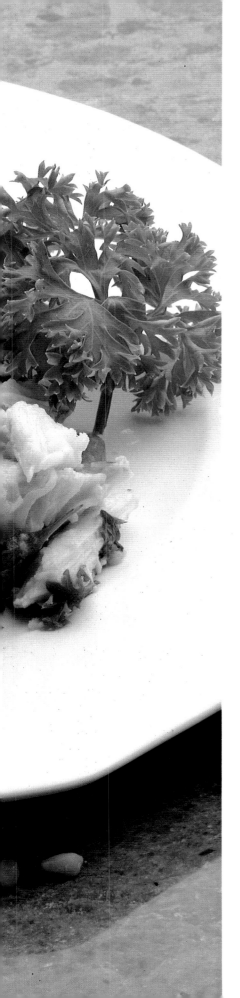

LOW-JOULE STARTERS

These tasty first course dishes will make a perfect start to any meal, without harming your waistline.

Crab Saute with Prosciutto

795 kilojoules/190 calories per serving

2 tspn lite margarine

1 cup freshly cooked crab meat

1 tblspn finely chopped spring onions (scallions)

1 tblspn finely chopped parsley

¼ tspn cracked black pepper

1 tblspn lemon juice

¼ tspn chilli paste or chopped fresh chilli

8 slices prosciutto

lemon for garnish

1 In a medium saucepan, heat margarine over moderate heat. Stir in the crab, spring onions, parsley, pepper, lemon juice and chilli paste and cook for 30 seconds.

2 Arrange 2 slices of prosciutto on each plate, then divide crab mixture between each plate and garnish with lemon if desired.

Serves 4

Asparagus Souffle

544 kilojoules/130 calories per serving

1.5kg (3lb) fresh asparagus, or 4 x 440g (14oz) cans asparagus tips, drained

300ml (½ pint) water, or liquid from asparagus cans

2 tpsn gelatine

2 cups plain low fat yoghurt

salt

pepper

4 egg-whites

1 Place asparagus in a steamer and cook over boiling water for about 8 minutes or until tender. Reserve cooking liquid.

2 Discard woody stalks. Mash asparagus with a fork and mix with the reserved liquid.

3 Dissolve gelatine in 2 tablespoons warm water. Add to asparagus mixture. Place mixture in a blender with yoghurt. Process until smooth. Season to taste with salt and pepper.

4 Beat egg-whites until stiff and fold into mixture. Rinse ramekins in cold water, shake dry. Pour mixture into ramekins and chill until firm. Serve garnished with asparagus tips.

Serves 8

Crab Saute with Prosciutto

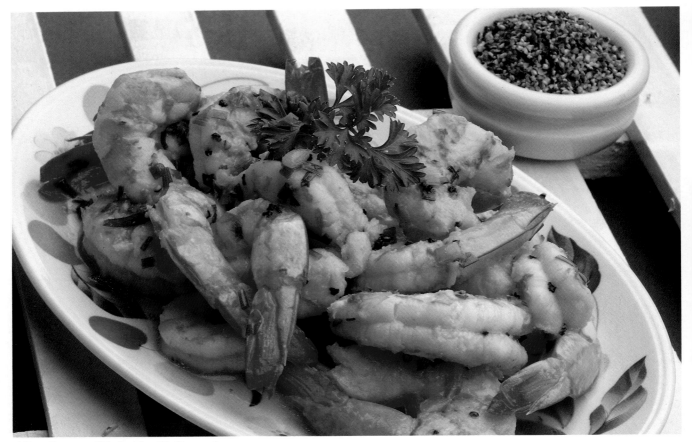

King Prawns (Shrimp) with Pernod

King Prawns (Shrimp) with Pernod

398 kilojoules/95 calories per serving

1 tblspn oil

2 cups green king prawns (shrimp), deveined and shelled, tails intact

1 clove garlic, crushed

2 tblspn finely chopped spring onions (scallions)

1 tblspn finely chopped chives

½ tspn cracked black pepper

2 tblspn pernod (or aniseed liqueur)

parsley sprig for garnish

1 In a large frying pan, heat the oil over moderate heat. Add the prawns, garlic, spring onions, chives, pepper and pernod.

2 Cook until prawns are no longer translucent, about 2 minutes, tossing frequently.

3 Serve immediately and garnish with parsley if desired.

Serves 4

Ricotta Roulade

649 kilojoules/155 calories per serving

410g (13oz) English spinach

2 tspn Dijon mustard

6 eggs, separated

salt

pepper

415g (13oz) fresh ricotta, mashed

1 bunch chives, finely chopped

1 lemon, cut into 8 wedges

1 Rinse spinach leaves thoroughly, place in a saucepan with only the water on the leaves and cook for 10 minutes. Drain, cool slightly. Chop very finely, place in a mixing bowl, add mustard and egg yolks. Season to taste with salt and pepper. Mix well.

2 Beat egg-whites until stiff, fold into spinach mixture. Line a baking sheet with greaseproof paper, top with mixture, cook in a 200°C (400°F) oven for 15-20 minutes.

3 Leave to cool for 3 minutes. Turn out gently onto a fresh sheet of greaseproof paper. Cover with mashed ricotta and chopped chives. Roll up gently with the help of the greaseproof paper and place in the oven for 5 minutes. Serve sliced, garnished with wedges of lemon.

Serves 8

Trout Timbale with Guacamole

1235 kilojoules/295 calories per serving

4 x 125g (4oz) skinless rainbow trout fillets

1 small ripe avocado, peeled, pitted and chopped

1 tspn very finely chopped red chilli

½ onion, peeled and very finely chopped

2 tblspn freshly squeezed lemon juice

¼ tspn white pepper

avocado and lemon for garnish

1 Line 4 x ½-cup capacity timbale tins with a trout fillet.

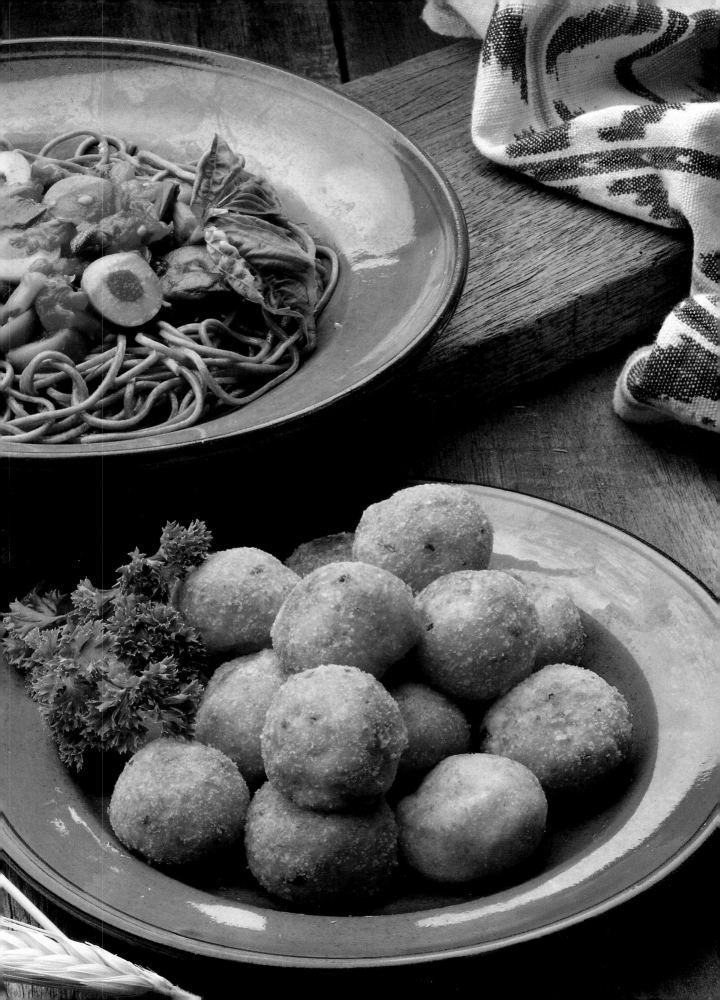

Stuffed Mushrooms

356 kilojoules/85 calories per serving

18 large mushrooms

1 tblspn freshly squeezed lemon juice

1 bunch coriander

¼ cup dry white wine

1 large onion, chopped

250g (½lb) spinach

15g (½oz) unsalted butter

salt

1 tblspn mustard seed oil

2 cloves garlic

100g (3½oz) mild chevre or other goat's cheese

1 Remove stalks from mushrooms, chop them finely in processor. Wipe mushroom caps with a damp cloth, sprinkle with lemon juice and set aside.

2 Reserving a few sprigs for garnish, separate coriander stems from leaves, chop both, keep separate.

3 Heat wine in a heavy saucepan, add onion, chopped coriander stalks, butter and mushroom stalks. Season to taste with salt. Cook, stirring constantly, until liquid evaporates.

4 Rinse spinach thoroughly and cook with only the water on the leaves until wilted. Drain and squeeze dry, chop finely.

5 Heat oil, cook garlic gently for 2-3 minutes. Add spinach and continue cooking for 4 minutes.

6 Combine spinach and garlic with mushroom mixture. Add goat's cheese, broken into small pieces and chopped coriander leaves. Mix well.

7 Using a teaspoon, mound mixture into mushroom caps. Place on a baking dish, bake 15-20 minutes in a 180°C (350°F) oven, or until golden brown on top. Garnish with coriander sprigs.

Serves 6

Garlic Goat's Cheese Toasts

795 kilojoules/190 calories per serving

8 radicchio leaves, washed and dried

½ cup cherry tomatoes, halved

1 cup watercress

8 slices bread, crusts removed

2 tspn crushed garlic

100g (3½oz) goat's cheese

50g (1¾oz) Philadelphia light cream cheese

½ tspn cracked black pepper

1 Arrange lettuce, tomatoes and watercress on 4 serving plates.

2 Toast the slices of bread on each side. Spread the crushed garlic very lightly on one side of each toast.

3 In a medium bowl, combine the goat's cheese, cream cheese and pepper, mix until smooth.

4 Spread each slice of toast with the cheese mixture and grill under low heat until cheese begins to brown.

5 Cut each slice into 2 triangles and divide toasts between the four plates of salad. Serve immediately.

Serves 4

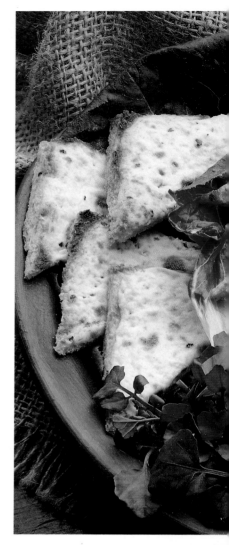

Snowpea Mousse

502 kilojoules/120 calories per serving

250g (½lb) snowpeas

150ml (¼ pint) water

2 tspn finely chopped onion

¼ cup chopped parsley

1 tblspn chopped fresh chives

½ sachet gelatine

salt

pepper

2 tspn freshly squeezed lemon juice

½ cup plain low fat yoghurt

1 egg-white, stiffly beaten

Melba toast to serve

1 Set aside 10 snowpeas for garnish. Bring water to a boil, pour most over peas and onions, leaving enough to dissolve gelatine in.

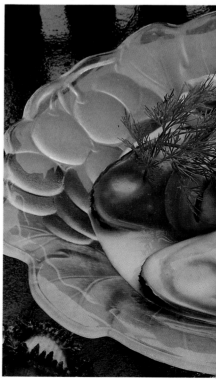

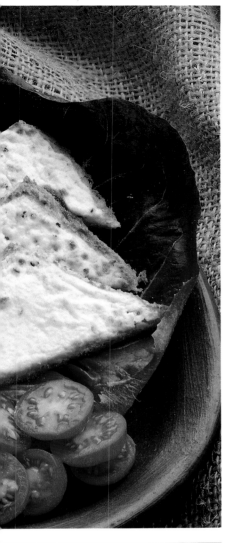

2 Cook snowpeas and onions until tender and process in processor or blender with cooking liquid. Sieve into a measuring jug. There should be about ¾ cup. Cool and add parsley and chives.

3 Dissolve gelatine in reserved warm water. Add to puree, season to taste with salt and freshly ground pepper, add lemon juice. Refrigerate.

4 When puree is on the point of setting, fold in yoghurt, followed by stiffly beaten egg-white.

5 Rinse five 100ml (3floz) ramekins with cold water. Shake dry, divide mixture evenly and refrigerate until set, at least 2 hours.

6 Lightly cook remaining snow-peas. Turn out moulds onto individual plates and garnish with snowpeas and serve with Melba toast.

Serves 5

Emerald Green Hot Garlic Dip

About 125 kilojoules/30 calories per tablespoon
About 63 kilojoules/15 calories per pita wedge

1 x 315g (10oz) package frozen spinach
12 cloves garlic
¼ cup milk
250g (½lb) package cream cheese, softened
salt
Tabasco sauce
60g (2oz) grated Cheddar cheese
2 pita loaves, halved horizontally, cut into 8 wedges each, toasted

1 Cook spinach according to directions. Drain, pressing down hard to express all moisture.

2 With machine running, drop garlic through feed tube of processor. Blend until finely chopped. Add spinach and milk. Combine well. Add cream cheese. Puree until smooth.

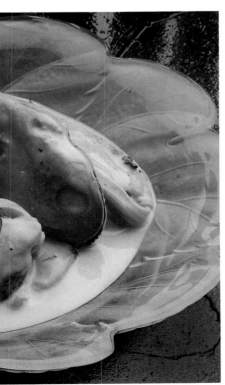

Top: Garlic Goat's Cheese Toasts.
Bottom: Mussels Cooked in Wine

3 Scrape mixture into a saucepan. Stir over medium heat until heated through. Season to taste with salt and Tabasco. Spoon into a heated serving dish, sprinkle with cheese. Serve with toasted pita wedges for dipping.

Makes about 2 cups

Mussels Cooked In Wine

1026 kilojoules/245 calories per serving
24 mussels, cleaned and debearded
2 cups dry white wine
1 onion, finely chopped
2 cloves garlic, crushed
2 tblspn chopped parsley
2 egg yolks
1 tblspn freshly squeezed lemon juice
1 tblspn Dijon mustard
3 tblspn oil
sprig of dill for garnish

1 In a large saucepan, combine the mussels, wine, onion, garlic and parsley over moderate heat. Bring to the boil, reduce heat, cover and simmer until mussel shells open, about 4 minutes, discard any that do not open.

2 Remove mussels with a slotted spoon, remove flesh from shells and reserve; discard the shells. Strain the mussel liquid and return to the pan.

3 Bring to the boil again and cook until it has reduced to ¼ cup, set aside and cool to room temperature.

4 In a medium bowl, whisk the egg yolks, lemon juice and mustard until creamy. Add the oil in droplets, while whisking, until mixture thickens.

5 Slowly whisk in the reduced mussel liquid, add the mussels and toss until well coated. Chill until ready to serve, garnish with fresh dill if desired.

Serves 4

SIDE SALADS

Add essential vitamins and minerals to your diet without adding kilojoules with these flavoursome side salads.

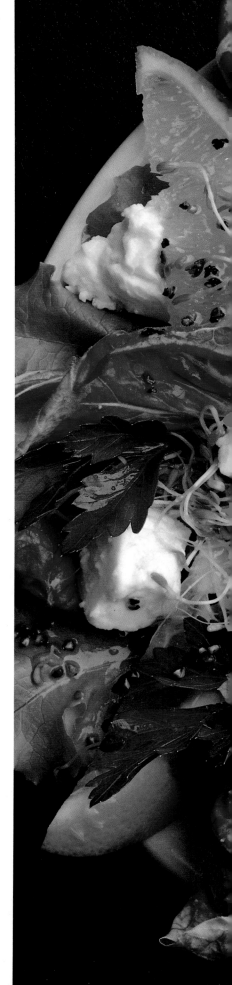

Tangy Cucumber and Coriander Salad

105 kilojoules/25 calories per serving

2 cucumbers, halved lengthwise, seeds removed

salt

¼ cup coarsely chopped fresh coriander

DRESSING

3 tblspn white wine vinegar

1 tspn castor sugar

1 tblspn finely shredded lemon zest

salt

1 Slice cucumber very thinly into half moons. Place in a colander, sprinkle with salt. Weigh down with a plate and a heavy object on top, eg some cans, stand 1 hour. Remove plate and weights, pat cucumber dry with paper towels. Place in a salad bowl.

2 To make dressing: Combine vinegar, sugar and lemon zest in a screwtop jar, season to taste with salt. Shake until well combined.

3 Add coriander to cucumber, toss salad with dressing to coat well. Cover, refrigerate for 2 hours. This salad actually improves in flavour under refrigeration, and can be kept refrigerated up to 2 days. In this case do not add coriander until just before serving.

Serves 4

Mixed Salad with Anchovy Pepper Dressing

879 kilojoules/210 calories per serving

1 radicchio lettuce

1 coral or butter lettuce

1 cup alfalfa sprouts

155g (5oz) feta cheese, crumbled

1 orange, cut into thin wedges

8 sprigs Italian parsley

1 tblspn olive oil

1 tspn cracked black pepper

2 tblspn freshly squeezed orange juice

3 anchovy fillets, mashed

1 Wash lettuce leaves and tear into pieces. Arrange the lettuce with the alfalfa, feta cheese, orange wedges and parsley, decoratively on a salad plate.

2 Pour over combined oil, pepper, orange juice and mashed anchovy fillets.

Serves 4

Mixed Salad with Anchovy Pepper Dressing

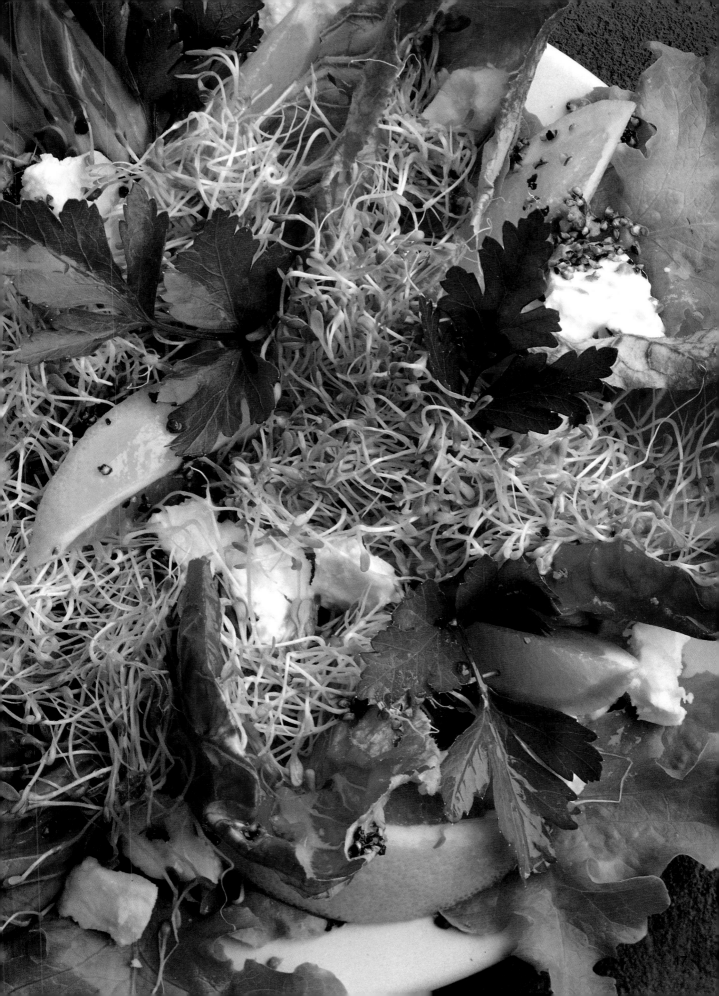

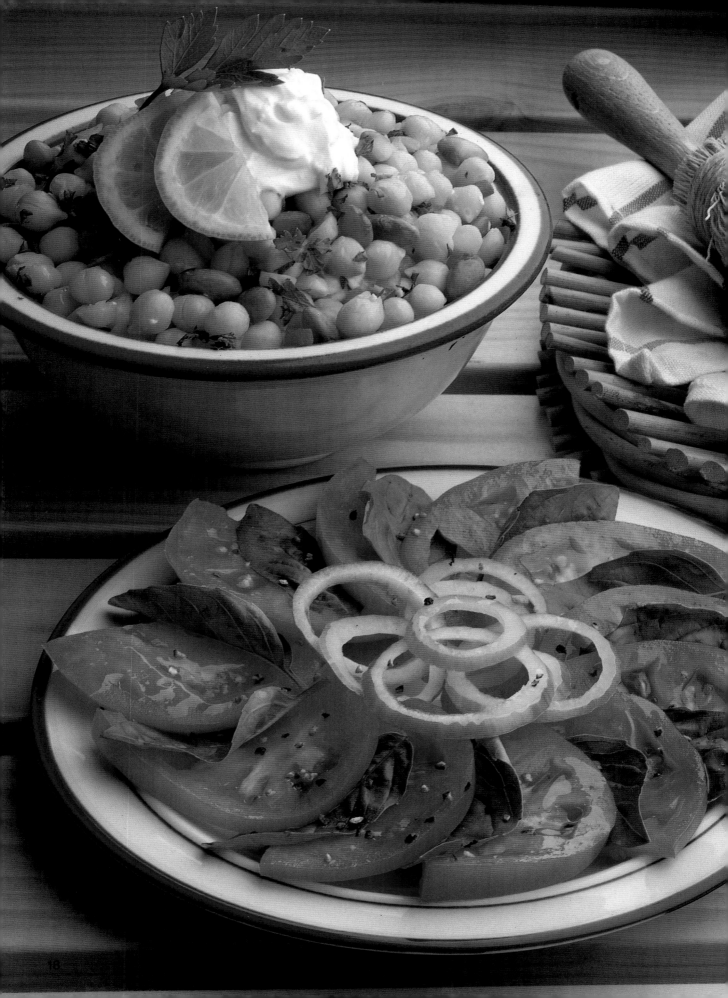

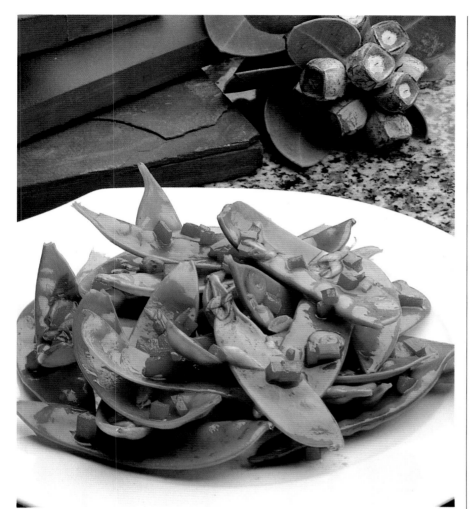

2 Place the onion rings in centre of each salad and pour over combined garlic, olive oil, lime juice and pepper.

Serves 4

Snowpeas with Walnut Vinaigrette

314 kilojoules/75 calories per serving

375g (¾lb) snowpeas, tops and tails cut off

¼ cup finely sliced spring onions (scallions)

¼ cup finely chopped red capsicum (pepper)

1 clove garlic, crushed

1 tblspn walnut oil

1 tblspn tarragon vinegar

1 In a large bowl, combine the snowpeas, spring onions, capsicum, garlic, walnut oil and vinegar.

2 Toss salad well and divide between four serving plates.

Serves 4

Fennel Salad

335 kilojoules/80 calories per serving

2 fennel bulbs

DRESSING

2 tblspn olive oil

1 tblspn freshly squeezed lemon juice

2 tblspn finely chopped parsley

1 tblspn finely chopped chives

salt

pepper

1 Cut fennel bulbs into 0.5cm (¼ in) slices crosswise. Separate rings, place in a salad bowl.

2 To make dressing: Combine oil, lemon juice, parsley and chives in a screwtop jar, shake until well combined. Season to taste with salt and freshly ground pepper. Shake again.

3 Pour dressing over fennel rings, toss to coat. Serve immediately.

Serves 4

Left: Top, Two Bean Salad with Light Cream Cheese and Lemon; bottom, Tomato Basil Salad. Above: Snowpeas with Walnut Vinaigrette

Two Bean Salad with Light Cream Cheese and Lemon

628 kilojoules/150 calories per serving

¾ cup dried chickpeas

¾ cup dried pinto beans

2 tblspn finely chopped parsley

2 tblspn finely chopped pimento

¼ cup freshly squeezed lemon juice

1 tblspn light cream cheese

1 In separate bowls, soak the chickpeas and pinto beans overnight in cold water. Drain beans and place in one large saucepan.

2 Cover beans with water and bring to the boil, reduce heat and simmer until beans are cooked, about 1¼ hours.

3 Drain beans and pour into a large bowl, stir in the parsley, pimento and lemon juice.

4 Pour salad into a serving bowl and serve with a tablespoon of the cream cheese. Garnish with lemon slices and parsley.

Serves 4

Tomato Basil Salad

335 kilojoules/80 calories per serving

2 large tomatoes, sliced

1 cup fresh basil leaves

1 red onion, peeled and sliced into rings

2 cloves garlic, crushed

2 tspn olive oil

1 tblspn freshly squeezed lime juice

½ tspn cracked black pepper

1 Cut each tomato slice in half and arrange alternately with basil leaves around the edge of each salad plate.

Zucchini (Courgette) and Tomato Salad

167 kilojoules/40 calories per serving

3 zucchini (courgette), sliced

2 spring onions (scallions), thinly sliced

salt

1 punnet cherry tomatoes, halved

2 tblspn chopped fresh basil

DRESSING

⅔ cup plain low fat yoghurt

1 clove garlic, crushed

2 tblspn chopped parsley

pepper

1 Combine zucchini and spring onions in a colander. Season to taste with salt, mix well, stand 15 minutes. Pat dry with paper towels. Place in a salad bowl.

2 To make dressing: Combine yoghurt, garlic and parsley in a small bowl, stir until smooth. Season to taste with freshly ground pepper.

3 Add tomatoes to salad bowl, pour over dressing, toss well to coat and sprinkle over chopped basil. Serve immediately or cover and refrigerate until ready to serve.

Serves 6

Apple and Celery Salad with Creamy Pecan Dressing

586 kilojoules/140 calories per serving

3 crisp Granny Smith apples

¼ cup freshly squeezed lemon juice

2 celery stalks, cut into 5cm (2in) julienne

8 lettuce leaves, torn into bite-size pieces

¼ cup coarsely chopped parsley

CREAMY PECAN DRESSING

½ cup plain low fat yoghurt

1 tblspn freshly squeezed lemon juice

1 tblspn honey

2 tblspn coarsely chopped pecan nuts

1 To make dressing: Combine yoghurt, lemon juice and honey in a small bowl. Whisk in pecan nuts, cover, refrigerate until ready to serve.

2 Core and thickly slice apples, do not peel. Drop into a bowl of water, accidulated with the lemon juice.

3 When ready to serve drain apples, combine in a bowl with celery. Add dressing, toss well to coat.

4 Divide lettuce among 4 plates, top with salad and sprinkle with parsley.

Serves 4

Sesame and Bean Sprout Salad

481 kilojoules/115 calories per serving

1 cup broccoli, broken into small pieces

1 cup bean sprouts

1 red capsicum (pepper), seeded and finely chopped

1 green capsicum (pepper), seeded and finely chopped

2 tspn honey

2 tspn soy sauce

1 tblspn oil

1 tspn sesame seeds

1 Bring a medium saucepan of water to the boil. Add broccoli and cook for 1 minute. Refresh broccoli under cold water and drain.

2 Arrange bean sprouts around the edge of each serving plate.

3 Mix together the broccoli, red and green capsicums, honey, soy sauce and oil. Toss well and arrange in the centre of the bean sprouts.

4 Sprinkle the sesame seeds over the top and serve.

Serves 4

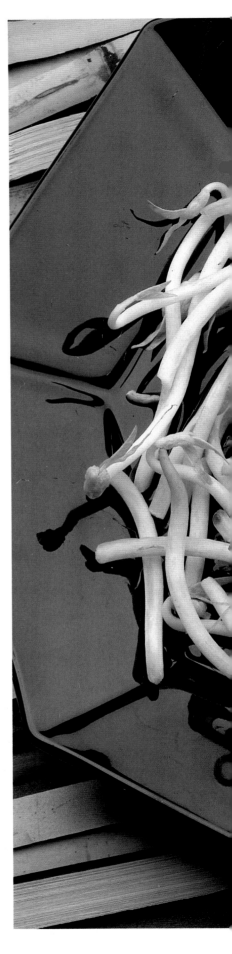

Sesame and Bean Sprout Salad

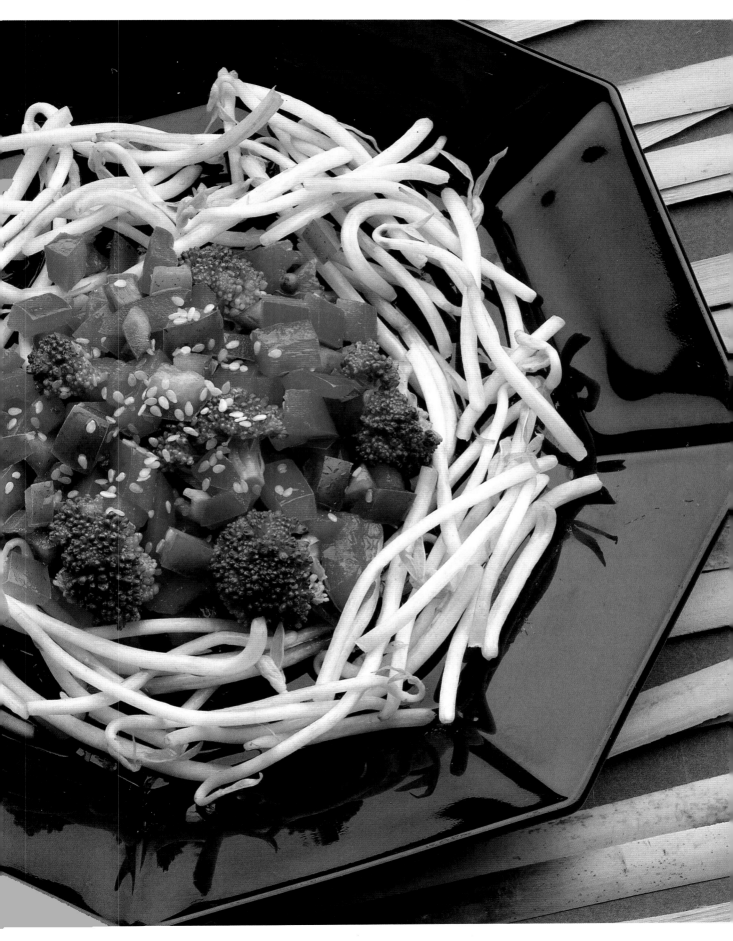

Witlof (Chicory, Belgian Endive) and Watercress Salad with Orange Dressing

105 kilojoules/25 calories per serving

3 heads witlof (UK chicory, US Belgian endive), leaves separated

185g (6oz) watercress, larger stems removed

ORANGE DRESSING

2 tspn mustard seed oil

2 tspn balsamic vinegar

2 tspn finely grated orange zest

salt

pepper

1 To make dressing: Combine oil, vinegar and orange zest in a screwtop jar, season to taste with salt and freshly ground pepper. Shake until well combined. Stand at room temperature for 30 minutes.

2 In a salad bowl combine witlof with watercress. Add dressing, toss well to coat. Serve immediately.

Serves 6

Tossed Egg and Mushroom Salad

921 kilojoules/220 calories per serving

1 coral lettuce or butter lettuce

1 cup cherry tomatoes

4 hard-boiled eggs, peeled and sliced

½ cup sliced button mushrooms

1 tblspn chopped chives

1 avocado, peeled and sliced

1 clove garlic, crushed

1 tblspn tarragon vinegar

2 tblspn orange juice

1 Wash the lettuce and tear into pieces. Arrange lettuce leaves, tomatoes, egg slices, mushrooms, chives and avocado in serving bowl.

2 Mix together the garlic, vinegar and orange juice and pour over salad just before serving.

Serves 4

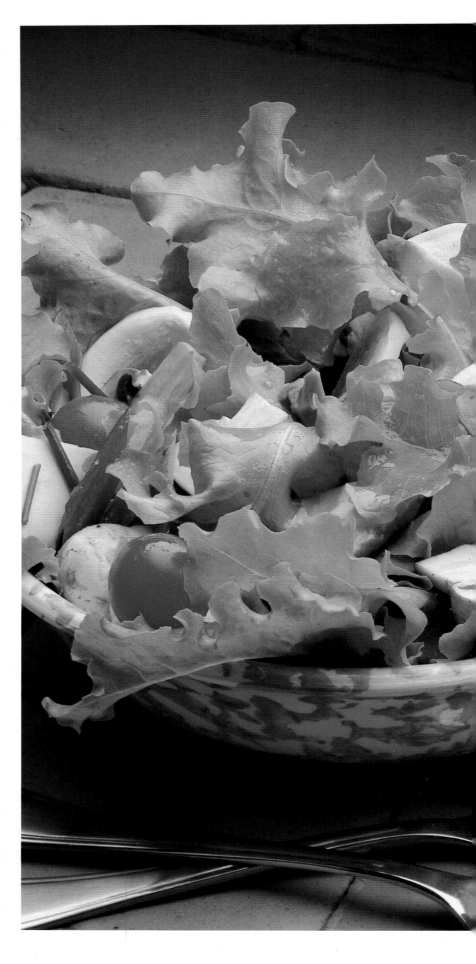

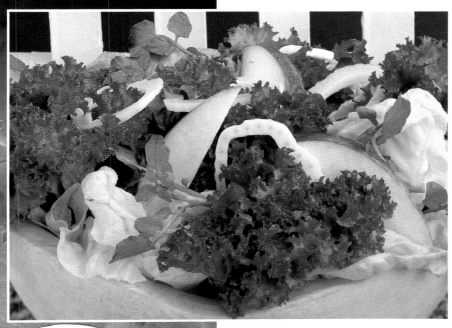

Tossed Egg and Mushroom Salad. Below: Tossed Salad with Lemon Dressing

Tossed Salad with Lemon Dressing

209 kilojoules/50 calories per serving

1 red lettuce (coral lettuce or radicchio)

1 butter lettuce

1 red apple, thinly sliced

1 fennel bulb, top cut off, finely sliced

1 cup watercress sprigs

juice of one lemon

1 Wash lettuce and tear leaves into pieces. Arrange lettuce, apple slices, fennel and watercress in a salad bowl.

2 Pour lemon juice over the top and serve immediately.

Serves 4

Arugula Salad with Warm Onion Vinaigrette

293 kilojoules/70 calories per serving

4 bunches arugula

pepper

2 tblspn finely chopped parsley

WARM ONION VINAIGRETTE

1½ tblspn walnut oil

½ small onion, very thinly sliced

salt

1½ tblspn red wine vinegar

1 To make Warm Onion Vinaigrette: Combine oil and onion in a small saucepan, add 2 teaspoons water and season to taste with salt. Cover, cook over very low heat for 5 minutes. Remove lid, cook until onion is tender, about a further 3 minutes. Add vinegar and 2 teaspoons water, cook until heated through, about 1 minute.

2 Place arugula in a salad bowl, pour over dressing, toss well to coat. Season with freshly ground pepper and sprinkle with parsley.

Serves 4

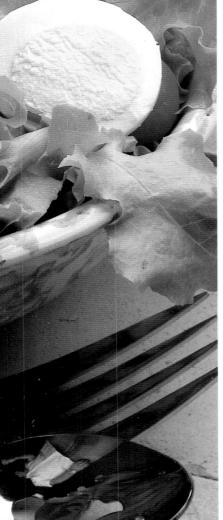

Green Salad with Mimosa Dressing

481 kilojoules/115 calories per serving

½ head curly endive, torn into bite-size pieces

½ cos lettuce, torn into bite-size pieces

MIMOSA DRESSING

3 tblspn olive oil

1 tblspn freshly squeezed lemon juice

1 tblspn white wine vinegar

1 hard-boiled egg, mashed with a fork

1 tblspn chopped fresh dill

salt

pepper

1 Place greens in a salad bowl.

2 To make dressing: Combine oil, lemon juice, vinegar, egg and dill in a screwtop jar. Shake until well combined. Season to taste with salt and freshly ground pepper. Shake again.

3 Pour dressing over salad greens, toss well to coat. Serve immediately.

Serves 6

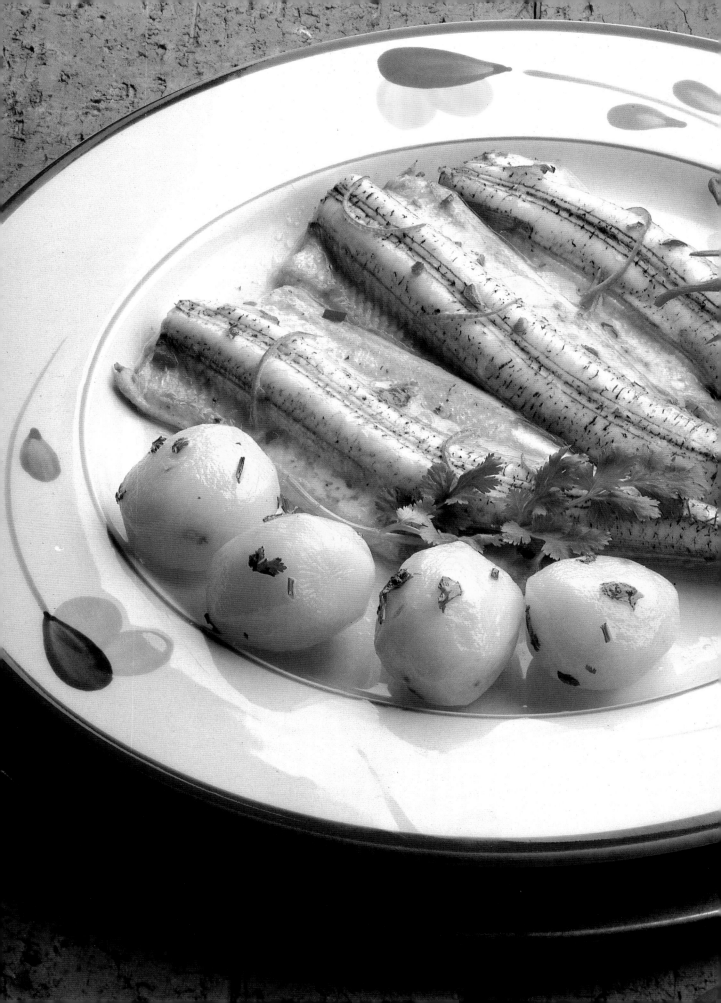

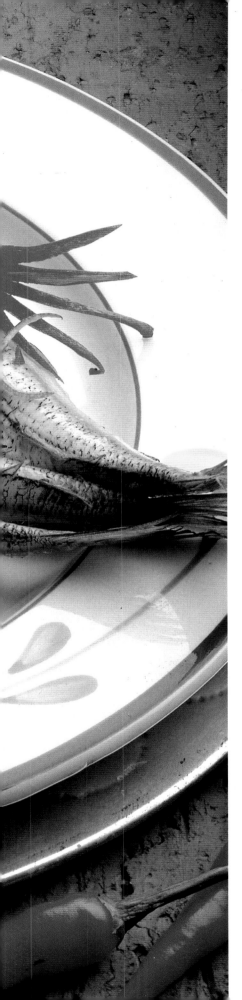

SUCCULENT SEAFOOD

Seafood is a wonderful food for people watching their weight. It's an excellent source of protein, vitamins and minerals, while low in kilojoules.

Garfish with Chilli, Lime and Coconut Sauce

1172 kilojoules/280 calories per serving

8 garfish (sea eel, eel), cleaned and scaled

1 tblspn oil

2 cloves garlic, crushed

1 cup coconut milk

½ cup freshly squeezed lime juice

½ tspn cracked black pepper

1 tblspn chopped fresh coriander

1 tspn finely chopped fresh chilli

boiled baby potatoes to serve

1 To prepare garfish: Cut off heads, make an incision from top to tail, being careful not to cut right through. Place fish cut side down and flatten out with palm of hand.

2 Heat the oil in a large frying pan over moderate heat. Add garlic, cook 1 minute. Add coconut milk, lime juice, pepper, coriander and chilli, bring to a boil, reduce heat, simmer 2 minutes.

3 Add garfish and poach for 3-4 minutes or until cooked through. Place fish on serving plates, pour pan juices over the top and serve with boiled baby potatoes.

Serves 4

Sole Seviche

691 kilojoules/165 calories per serving

500g (1lb) sole (Dover sole, flounder) fillets, cut into 2.5cm (1in) strips

16 lettuce leaves

1 small Spanish onion, thinly sliced, rings separated

MARINADE

juice of 8 limes

juice of 2 lemons

juice of 2 oranges

2 tblspn chopped fresh coriander

1 clove garlic, crushed

1 tspn sambal oelek (see note)

2 tblspn sugar

salt

pepper

1 Place sole strips in a dish large enough to hold fish in one layer.

2 Combine lime, lemon and orange juice, coriander, garlic, sambal oelek and sugar in a bowl. Add salt and freshly ground pepper to taste. Stir well.

3 Pour marinade over fish, cover, refrigerate at least 4 hours, or until fish is opaque.

4 Divide lettuce among 4 serving plates, spoon seviche on top, scatter with onion rings. Serve cold.

Note: Sambal Oelek is a chilli paste, available in Asian food stores.

Serves 4

Garfish with Chilli, Lime and Coconut Sauce

Scallop and Prawn (Shrimp) Kebabs with Mango Marinade

921 kilojoules/220 calories per serving, 3 each

1 large mango, peeled and pitted, flesh chopped

2 tblspn freshly squeezed lime juice

18 scallops, deveined

18 green king prawns (shrimp), deveined, peeled, tails intact

½ tspn cracked black pepper

1 choko (chayote), cut into 2cm (¾in) cubes

12 wooden skewers, soaked in water for 1 hour

1 In a food processor or blender, puree the mango flesh and lime juice until smooth.

2 In a medium bowl, combine the scallops, prawns, mango sauce and pepper, cover and refrigerate for 1 hour.

3 Bring a large saucepan of water to the boil, add the choko pieces and cook for 4 minutes, remove with a slotted spoon and refresh under cold water.

4 Thread the scallops, alternating with the prawns and choko pieces on the skewers.

5 Brush with the mango marinade and grill under a moderate heat for 1-2 minutes each side. Serve immediately.

Makes 12

Poached Salmon with Asparagus Topping

1465 kilojoules/350 calories per serving

1 tblspn oil

2 cloves garlic, crushed

3 spring onions (scallions), sliced

1 cup tinned asparagus, drained and chopped

4 salmon cutlets, 150-200g (5-6oz) each

1½ tblspn Dijon mustard

¼ cup grated mature cheese

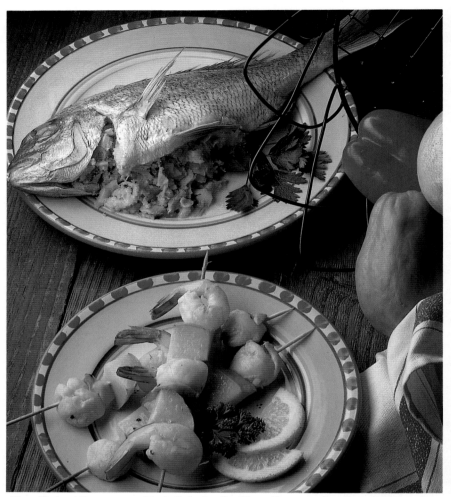

Top: Baked Snapper with Artichoke Stuffing. Bottom: Scallop and Prawn (Shrimp) Kebabs with Mango Marinade

1 Heat the oil in a medium frying pan over moderate heat. Add the garlic and spring onions, cook for 1 minute. Remove frying pan from heat and stir in the asparagus, set aside.

2 Place the salmon cutlets in a lightly greased baking dish and bake in moderate oven for 15 minutes.

3 Spread the top side of each cutlet with the mustard, then spoon the asparagus mixture on top. Sprinkle with cheese and return to the oven for 5-10 minutes or until cheese has melted.

4 Serve with fresh blanched vegetables.

Serves 4

Sicilian Ling Fillet and Artichokes

1110 kilojoules/265 calories per serving

1½ tblspn olive oil

500g (1lb) ling (pike, freshwater perch) fillets, cut into 3cm (1¼in) strip)

1 onion, chopped

4 cloves garlic, chopped

1 cup dry red wine

800g (26oz) canned tomatoes, chopped, with juice

6 black olives, thickly sliced

½ tspn capers

¼ tspn chilli flakes

4 artichoke hearts, drained, quartered

1 Heat olive oil in a heavy frying pan, add ling, sear over high heat for 1 minute each side, remove from pan, set aside.

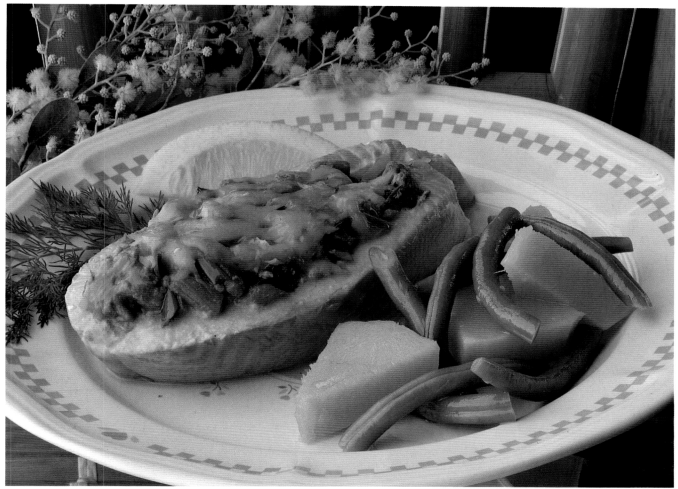

Poached Salmon with Asparagus Topping

2 Reduce heat to medium high, add onion to pan, saute until light golden, about 5 minutes. Add garlic, cook a further minute.

3 Add wine, cook until most liquid has evaporated, about 5 minutes. Add tomatoes and their juice, olives, capers and chilli flakes. Bring to a boil, cook until reduced by half, about a further 5 minutes.

4 Reduce heat to medium, stir artichokes into the sauce, arrange fish on top. Cover pan, cook until fish is opaque, about 8-10 minutes. Remove fish to a heated serving dish.

5 Increase heat to high, cook until sauce thickens. Remove artichokes with a slotted spoon, add to fish, pour sauce over. Serve hot.

Serves 4

Baked Snapper with Artichoke Stuffing

837 kilojoules/200 calories per serving

2 tblspn lite margarine

1 onion, peeled and chopped

2 cloves garlic, crushed

½ red capsicum (pepper), seeded and chopped

1 cup artichoke hearts, drained and finely chopped

2 tblspn freshly squeezed lime juice

1 tblspn chopped fresh parsley

¼ cup dried breadcrumbs

2 snapper (red mullet, black sea bass), head and tail left on

2 tblspn freshly squeezed lemon juice

3 tblspn freshly squeezed lime juice

¼ cup dry white wine

parsley sprig for garnish

1 Heat the margarine in a medium frying pan over moderate heat. Add the onions, garlic and red capsicum, cook for 3 minutes. Stir in the artichoke, lime juice, parsley and breadcrumbs.

2 Fill the fish cavity with the artichoke mixture and secure cavity with toothpicks.

3 Lightly grease a flat baking dish, large enough to hold the fish, and pour combined lemon, lime juice and wine over the fish.

4 Bake, basting frequently with the pan juices until fish is cooked, 30-40 minutes. Serve fish immediately, garnished with fresh parsley.

Each fish serves 2

Perch with Vegetables and Sour Cream Sauce

1130 kilojoules/270 calories per serving

1 tspn unsalted butter, melted

1 bunch spring onions (scallions), cut into 2.5cm (1in) lengths

salt

pepper

juice of 1 lemon

4 deep sea perch (sea bass, catfish) fillets, 155g (5oz) each

4 medium tomatoes, chopped

½ cup chopped button mushrooms

½ cup chopped continental parsley

150ml (¼ pint) dry white wine

½ cup light sour cream

1 Brush ovenproof dish, large enough to hold fillets in one layer, with melted butter. Arrange spring onions in the dish. Season with a little salt.

2 Season fillets with salt and freshly ground pepper to taste, sprinkle with lemon juice. Arrange fillets on top of spring onions, sprinkle with tomatoes, mushrooms and parsley.

3 Pour over wine, cover with foil, cook in a 180° (350°F) oven for 20 minutes, or until fish is cooked through. Tip dish and pour liquid out of one corner into a saucepan. Keep fish warm.

4 Add sour cream to saucepan, bring to a boil, cook until sauce is slightly reduced and coats a spoon.

5 Arrange fish fillets onto heated plates, spoon over vegetables and pour over sauce. Serve immediately.

Serves 4

Poached Jewfish with Julienne Vegetables

1130 kilojoules/270 calories per serving

1 tblspn oil

¼ cup semi-sweet white wine

1 choko (chayote), cut into thin strips

155g (5oz) pumpkin, peeled and cut into thin strips

1 red capsicum (pepper), seeded and cut into thin strips

¼ tspn cracked black pepper

½ cup semi-sweet white wine, extra

¼ cup freshly squeezed lime juice

2 tblspn soy sauce

3 tblspn Worcestershire sauce

½ cup water

4 jewfish (turbot, rockfish) fillets, 155g (5oz) each, cut into rectangles

watercress sprigs to garnish

1 Heat the oil and wine in a large frying pan over moderate heat. Add the choko, pumpkin, red capsicum and pepper and stir over heat for 2 minutes.

2 Remove vegetables with a slotted spoon and keep warm in an oven-proof dish in a low oven.

3 Add the extra wine, lime juice, soy sauce, Worcestershire sauce and water to the frying pan. Bring to the boil, reduce heat to a simmer, add the jewfish pieces.

4 Cover and cook fish for 4 minutes on each side or until cooked through.

5 Arrange vegetables on each serving plate, place jewfish fillets on top and garnish with watercress sprigs.

Serves 4

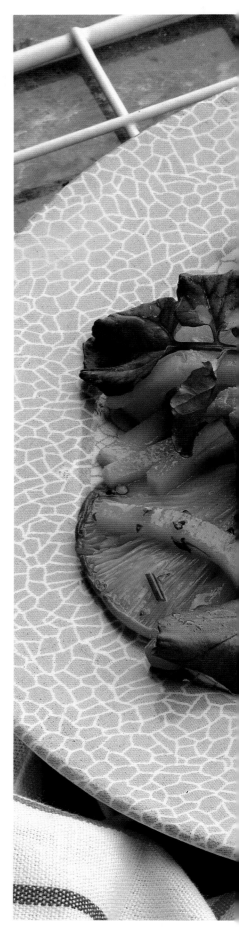

Poached Jewfish with Julienne Vegetables

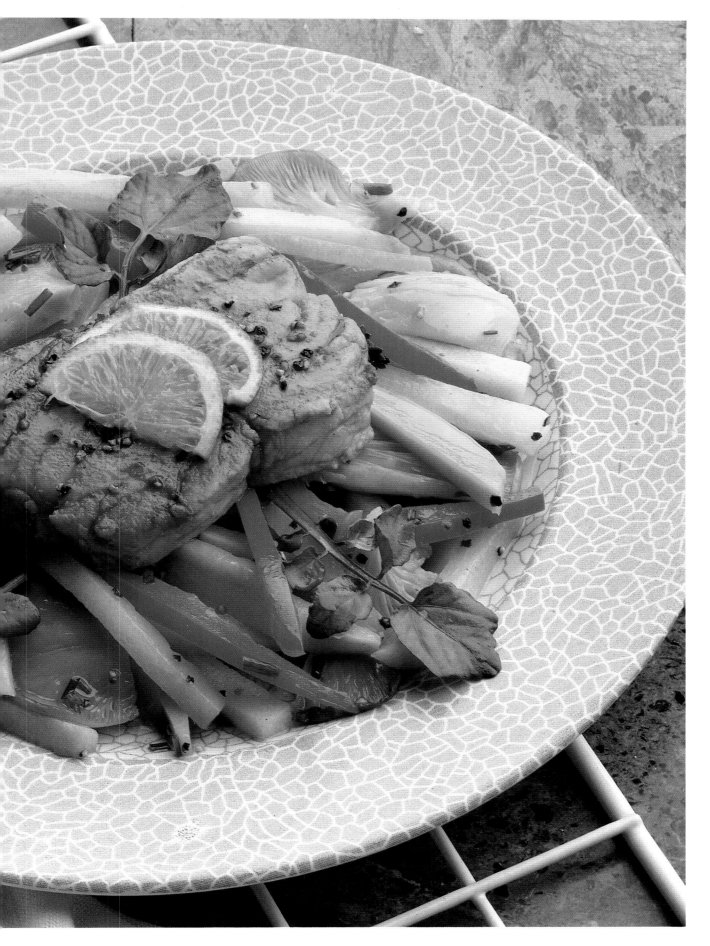

Snapper and Spinach Salad with Mango

1047 kilojoules/250 calories per serving

2 tspn oil

3 tblspn soy sauce

1 tblspn honey

¼ tspn cracked black pepper

¼ cup red wine vinegar

4 snapper (monkfish, tile) fillets, 155g (5oz) each, cut into 2cm (¾in) cubes

1 red capsicum (pepper), seeded and cut into strips

8 spinach leaves, torn into bite-size pieces

1 mango, pitted and peeled, cut into cubes

1 Heat the oil in a large frying pan over moderate heat. Add the soy sauce, honey, pepper and red wine vinegar, cook for 1 minute.

2 Add the fish pieces and cook for 3-5 minutes, or until cooked through. Remove fish with a slotted spoon and set aside.

3 Add the red capsicum to the frying pan and cook for 3 minutes, stirring occasionally.

4 Arrange the spinach leaves, mango, red capsicum and fish pieces in a serving bowl.

Serves 4

Seafood Sausages with Tomato Sauce

879 kilojoules/210 calories per serving

8 spinach leaves

¼ bunch watercress

1 tblspn lite margarine

625g (1lb 4oz) boneless fish fillets, skin removed

1 egg-white

3 tblspn skim milk

¼ tspn ground nutmeg

1 tblspn chopped chives

2 tblspn freshly squeezed lime juice

½ cup tomato puree

2 tspn tomato paste

2 drops Tabasco sauce

1 Cut off and discard the spinach and watercress stems, wash the leaves and pat them dry, then chop finely.

2 Melt the margarine in a large frying pan over moderate heat, add the spinach and watercress and toss for 1 minute. Transfer mixture into a bowl and refrigerate for 1 hour.

3 Puree the fish in a food processor or blender, for 1 minute. Add the egg-white and process a further 30 seconds. Add the milk gradually while processor is running, then add the spinach and watercress, process a further 1 minute.

4 Place mousse mixture into a bowl, cover and refrigerate until cold. Remove cover and mix in nutmeg, chives and lime juice.

5 Cut 8 foil rectangles, about 25x12cm (10x5in) and lightly grease each one. Place teaspoons of mixture along each foil rectangle, roll up into a sausage shape.

6 In a large frying pan heat enough water to cover the foil sausages. When simmering, add the sausages and cook for 6 minutes. Remove with a slotted spoon, set aside.

7 Heat the tomato puree, tomato paste and Tabasco in a medium saucepan, over moderate heat, until warmed through. Pour sauce on each serving plate, unwrap sausages and serve on top of sauce. Makes 8 sausages.

Serves 4

Atlantic Salmon with Garlic Sauce

984 kilojoules/235 calories per serving

2 tblspn olive oil

4 Atlantic salmon (salmon) steaks, 155g (5oz) each

1 red chilli, very thinly sliced

16 cloves garlic, finely chopped

½ cup finely chopped dill

salt

pepper

2 cups fish stock, made from non-oily fish and bones

sprigs of dill for garnish

1 Heat oil in a frying pan large enough to hold fish in one layer. Add garlic, chilli and dill, saute 1 minute. Arrange fish on top, season to taste with salt and freshly ground pepper.

2 Add stock, bring to a simmer, basting fish from time to time. Cover, cook over very low heat until fish is opaque, about 8 minutes.

3 Transfer fish to a heated serving dish with a slotted spoon. Remove skin, keep warm.

4 Boil pan juices over high heat until half a cup of liquid remains, about 10 minutes. Pour over fish, serve warm or at room temperature, garnished with dill sprigs.

Serves 4

Prawn (Shrimp) Curry for Springtime

837 kilojoules/200 calories per serving

1 tblspn ghee

1 tblspn safflower oil

1 large onion, chopped

2 stalks celery, chopped

2 red capsicum (peppers), cut into 1cm (½in) cubes

1½ tblspn curry powder

2 cups chopped, peeled and seeded cucumbers

425g (13½oz) can Italian peeled tomatoes, chopped, with juice

1 cup degreased chicken stock

750g (1½lb) uncooked prawns (shrimp), shelled and deveined

¼ cup unsweetened dessicated coconut

1 tblspn freshly squeezed lemon juice

salt

pepper

1 Heat ghee and oil in a frying pan, add onion, celery and capsicum, saute over medium high heat until softened, about 5 minutes.

2 Add curry powder, reduce heat to medium, cook 2 minutes, stirring constantly. Add cucumbers, cook 3 minutes, stirring constantly.

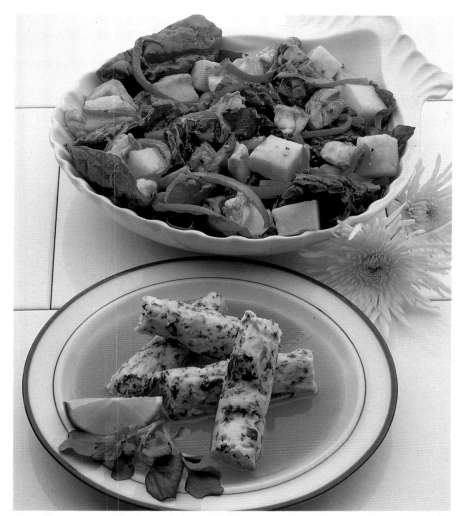

Top: Snapper and Spinach Salad with Mango. Bottom: Seafood Sausages with Tomato Sauce

3 Add tomatoes and juice and chicken stock. Bring to a boil, reduce heat, add prawns. Cook until prawns have become opaque, about 3-5 minutes.

4 Remove from heat, stir in coconut and lemon juice. Season to taste with salt and freshly ground pepper. Serve immediately.

Serves 6

Pepper Gemfish Fillets

628 kilojoules/150 calories per serving

6 gemfish (sea bream, pompano) fillets, 125g (4oz) each

¼ cup cracked black peppercorns

¾ cup vegetable stock

1 tspn chopped fresh marjoram

1½ tblspn unsalted butter, softened

marjoram sprigs for garnish

MARINADE

½ cup freshly squeezed lemon juice

½ cup red wine vinegar

2 cloves garlic, crushed

1 tblspn sugar

salt

1 To make marinade: Combine lemon juice, vinegar, garlic, sugar and salt to taste in a dish large enough to hold fish in one layer. Stir well to combine.

2 Arrange fish fillets in the dish, spoon over marinade. Cover, refrigerate at least 4 hours, or preferably overnight, turning fillets over once.

3 Remove fillets from marinade, coat with peppercorns, pressing in well with your hands. Place on a lightly oiled griller tray, cook under a pre-heated grill about 8 minutes, turning once, or until fish flakes easily when prodded. Place on a heated platter, keep warm.

4 Meanwhile, strain marinade into a saucepan, add stock and marjoram. Cook over medium heat until reduced to half a cup, about 5 minutes.

5 Whisk softened butter into the sauce, pour sauce over fillets. Serve immediately, garnished with sprigs of marjoram.

Serves 6

Mussels with Vegetable Julienne

440 kilojoules/105 calories per serving

¼ cup julienne of carrots

¼ cup julienne of celery

¼ cup chopped parsley

4 cloves garlic, chopped

½ cup dry white wine

½ cup water

2kg (4lb) mussels, scrubbed, beards removed

2 spring onions (scallions), sliced into thin rings

salt

pepper

1 Combine carrots, celery, parsley, garlic, wine and water in a large saucepan. Bring to a boil, reduce heat to a simmer, cook 3 minutes.

2 Add mussels, increase heat to high. Cover, steam mussels, shaking the pan from side to side over the heat, until mussels have opened, about 5 minutes. Remove open mussels, cook remaining mussels a few minutes longer. Discard any mussels which have not opened after additional cooking.

3 Divide mussels among 4 heated deep bowls. Stir spring onions into broth, season to taste with salt and freshly ground pepper. Ladle over mussels, serve hot.

Serves 4

POULTRY DISHES

Lean poultry without skin is low in fat but rich in niacin, one of the B vitamins, which is essential for good health.

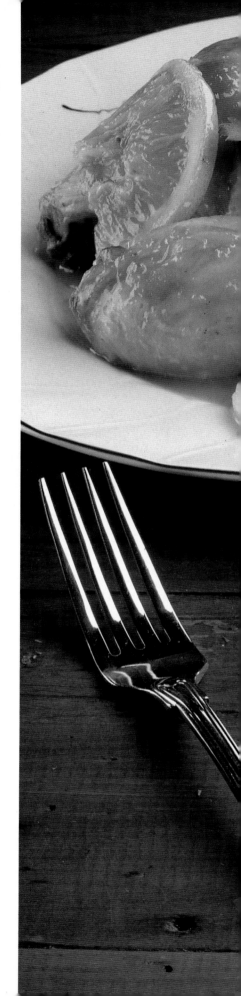

Baked Chicken Pieces with Orange Sauce

1403 kilojoules/335 calories per serving

1 tblspn butter

3 chicken Marylands, skin removed, broken into pieces

½ cup sweet white wine

½ cup freshly squeezed orange juice

½ orange, cut into thin slices

¼ cup apple juice

2 tblspn freshly squeezed lime juice

1 tblspn honey

1 Heat the butter in a large frying pan over moderate heat. Add the chicken pieces and cook for 4 minutes, stirring constantly.

2 Remove chicken, place in a baking dish and cook in a moderate oven for 20 minutes or until cooked through.

3 Meanwhile, add the wine, orange juice, oranges, apple juice, lime juice and honey to frying pan and bring liquid to the boil, reduce heat and simmer for 5-7 minutes or until sauce thickens slightly.

4 Remove chicken from oven and add to the frying pan. Turn chicken to cover in sauce, pour chicken and orange sauce into serving dish.

Serves 4

Chicken Medallions with Pimento Sauce

921 kilojoules/220 calories per serving

4 chicken fillets

2 tblspn freshly squeezed lemon juice

8 spinach leaves, stems removed

1 cup pimentos, drained and chopped

1 medium onion, chopped

2 tblspn tomato puree

1 tblspn natural yoghurt

4 watercress sprigs

1 Brush chicken fillets with lemon juice and cut into 4 neat rectangles. Lay 2 spinach leaves on each fillet and roll up into a sausage shape. Wrap each roll in foil.

2 Bake chicken rolls in a moderate oven for 20-25 minutes.

3 Meanwhile, make the sauce: Puree the pimentos with the onions and tomato puree until smooth. Divide sauce into two bowls. Stir the yoghurt into one bowl to make a pale pink sauce.

4 Carefully spoon equal amounts of each sauce on each plate.

5 Unwrap the chicken rolls and slice with a sharp knife. Arrange the chicken slices decoratively on top of the sauce. Garnish with fresh watercress sprigs.

Serves 4

Top: Baked Chicken Pieces with Orange Sauce. Bottom: Chicken Medallions with Pimento Sauce

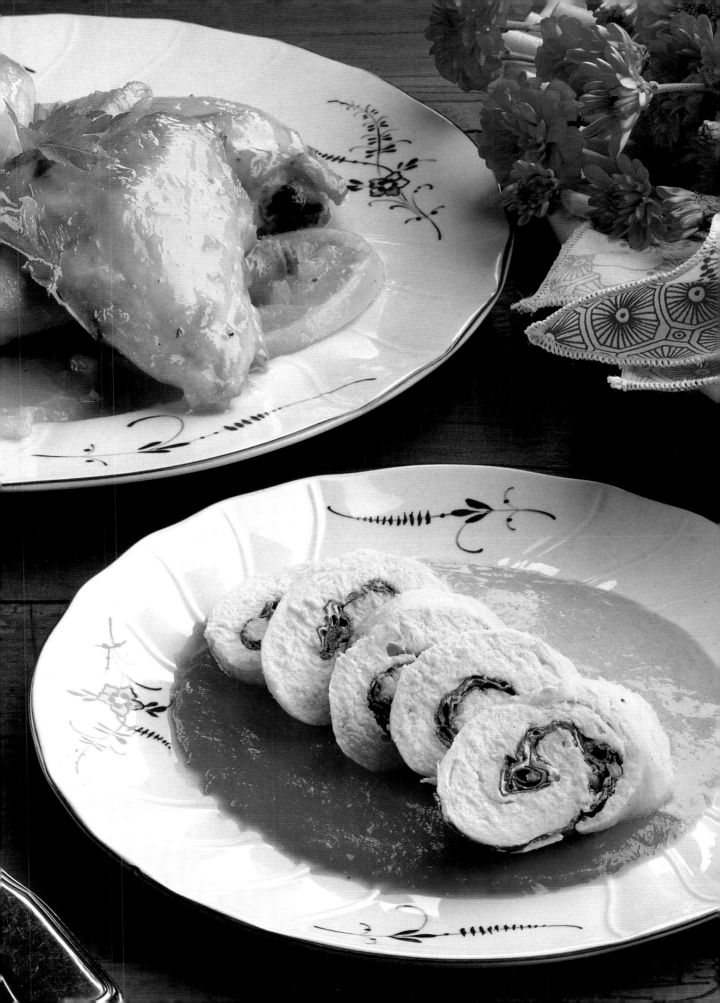

Chicken Curry with Yoghurt

879 kilojoules/210 calories per serving

4 skinless, boneless chicken breast halves
1 cup dry white wine
1 small leek
1 bay leaf
4 sprigs parsley
1 carrot, thickly sliced
2 tblspn safflower oil
2 cloves garlic, finely chopped
2 tblspn grated fresh ginger
2 tblspn curry powder
3 tomatoes, peeled, chopped
1 fennel bulb, chopped
1 Granny Smith apple, cored, coarsely chopped
2 stalks celery, sliced
2 large zucchini (courgette), sliced
2 large carrots, sliced
2 large onions, chopped
1 cup plain yoghurt
salt
pepper

1 Combine chicken, wine, leek, bay leaf, parsley and carrot in a saucepan, add 2 cups of water. Bring to a boil, reduce heat to a simmer, cover, cook about 10 minutes, or until chicken is tender.

2 Measure 1½ cups of the liquid, reserve to make the curry, leave chicken to cool in remaining poaching liquid.

3 Heat oil in a casserole, add garlic and ginger, saute until softened, about 2 minutes. Add curry powder, tomatoes, fennel, apple, zucchini, celery, carrots, onions and the reserved liquid.

4 Bring to a boil, reduce heat to a simmer, cook uncovered until sauce is thick, about 1 hour. Add a little more poaching liquid if sauce becomes too thick.

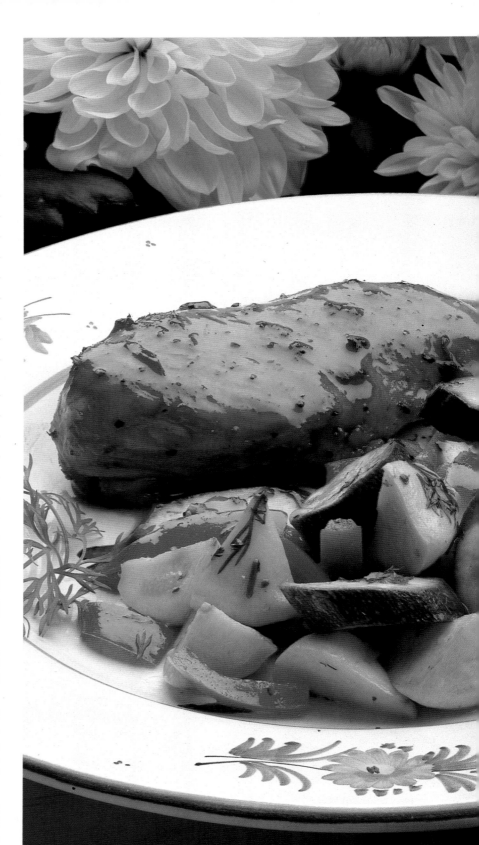

Left: Chicken Breast with Tricolour Vegetables. Below: Chicken Teriyaki with Yoghurt Chilli Sauce

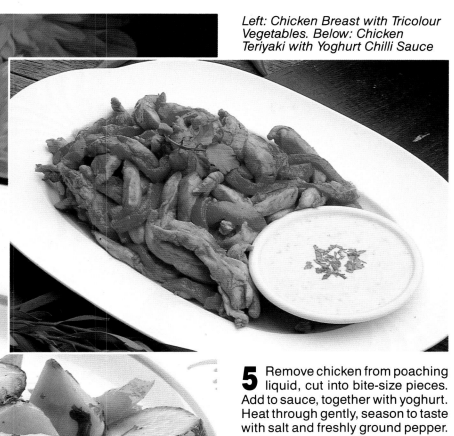

2 Add the chicken breasts and vegetables and cook the chicken for 3 minutes each side. Add the dill and pepper, toss vegetables and remove them with a slotted spoon, place in a warm oven.

3 Add the honey, tamari and tomato paste to the frying pan increase the heat and cook for 2 minutes turning the chicken frequently to coat well.

4 Serve chicken with the pan sauce and place vegetables on the side of plate.

Serves 4

Chicken Teriyaki with Yoghurt Chilli Sauce

1298 kilojoules/310 calories per serving

1 tblspn oil

3 tblspn soy sauce

3 tblspn Worcestershire sauce

2 tblspn red wine vinegar

¾ cup dry sherry

2 tblspn brown sugar

2 cloves garlic, crushed

4 single chicken breast fillets, cut into thin strips

4 pimentos, cut into thin strips

½ cup natural low fat yoghurt

1 tblspn freshly squeezed lime juice

¼ tspn sambal oelek (chilli paste)

1 Heat the oil in a large frying pan over moderate heat. Add the soy sauce, Worcestershire sauce, red wine vinegar, dry sherry, brown sugar and garlic and cook for 2 minutes.

2 Stir in the chicken pieces and pimentos, cook until chicken is cooked through and sauce thickened slightly.

3 To make yoghurt sauce: Mix the yoghurt with the lime juice and sambal oelek. Garnish with fresh chopped herbs if desired.

Serves 4

5 Remove chicken from poaching liquid, cut into bite-size pieces. Add to sauce, together with yoghurt. Heat through gently, season to taste with salt and freshly ground pepper.

Serves 6

Chicken Breast with Tricolour Vegetables

1089 kilojoules/260 calories per serving

1 tblspn olive oil

3 tblspn red wine vinegar

3 tblspn red wine

2 tblspn Worcestershire sauce

4 single chicken breasts

4 zucchini (courgette), sliced

1 cup yellow baby squash, cut into quarters

1 red capsicum (pepper), seeded, cut into small thin strips

1 tblspn chopped dill

½ tspn cracked black pepper

1 tblspn honey

1 tblspn tamari sauce

2 tspn tomato paste

1 Heat the oil in a large frying pan over moderate heat. Add the red wine vinegar, wine and Worcestershire sauce, cook 1 minute.

Turkey Breasts with Citrus Sauce

1570 kilojoules/375 calories per serving

1½ cups degreased chicken stock

1 tblspn chopped fresh rosemary

plain flour

salt

pepper

375g (¾lb) turkey breast, cut into 12 slices

¼ cup olive oil

½ small onion, thinly sliced

¾ cup freshly squeezed grapefruit juice

½ cup freshly squeezed orange juice

1 tspn chopped fresh thyme

¼ tspn chilli powder

1 Combine chicken stock and rosemary in a small saucepan. Bring to a boil, reduce heat to a simmer, cook 5 minutes, set aside.

2 Season some plain flour with salt and freshly ground pepper. Use to dust turkey slices, shake to remove excess.

3 Heat 1 tablespoon of the olive oil in a frying pan, add 4 turkey slices, saute until golden, about 4 minutes, turning once. Remove to a warm platter. Repeat the process with remaining oil and turkey, cover, set aside.

4 Add onion to frying pan, reduce heat, saute until softened, about 5 minutes. Add grapefruit and orange juice. Increase heat, bring to a boil, scraping up any browned bits from the bottom.

5 Strain chicken stock into the pan, discard rosemary. Add thyme and chilli powder, boil until liquid is reduced to 2 cups.

6 Reduce heat, return turkey slices to the pan, cook until heated through, about 2 minutes. With a slotted spoon transfer turkey to a heated serving platter. Check seasoning of the sauce, pour over turkey. Serve immediately.

Serves 6

Chicken Breasts with Spring Onions (Scallions)

1214 kilojoules/290 calories per serving

4 skinless, boneless chicken breast halves, 155g (5oz) each

flour

3 tblspn unsalted butter

1 cup chopped spring onion (scallion)

2 small cloves garlic, finely chopped

½ cup dry white wine

salt

pepper

1 tblspn freshly squeezed lemon juice

2 tspn grated lemon zest

1 tblspn chopped parsley

2 tblspn breadcrumbs

1 Place chicken breasts between layers of greaseproof paper, beat to an even thickness. Dust with flour, shake off excess.

2 Melt 2 tablespoons of the butter in a frying pan, add chicken, saute until golden brown on both sides, about 6 minutes, turning once. Remove from pan, set aside.

3 Reduce heat, add spring onion and garlic, cook until softened, about 5 minutes. Add wine, bring to a boil, cook until reduced by half, scraping up any browned bits from the bottom.

4 Pour half the sauce in a lightly greased baking dish, just large enough to hold the chicken in one layer. Add chicken, season to taste with salt and freshly ground pepper, sprinkle with lemon juice.

5 Spoon over remaining sauce, sprinkle with zest, parsley and breadcrumbs. Dot with remaining tablespoon butter.

6 Bake in a 200°C (400°F) oven until chicken is cooked through, about 15 minutes. Serve immediately.

Serves 4

Chicken Pieces with Mushrooms and Basil

963 kilojoules/230 calories per serving

1 tblspn olive oil

4 chicken breast fillets, cut into strips

1 tblspn butter

2 leeks, sliced, white part only

1 cup button mushrooms, sliced

½ cup drained and sliced sun-dried tomatoes

2 tblspn red wine vinegar

3 tblspn freshly squeezed lime juice

½ tspn chopped fresh chilli

1 tblspn chopped red or green basil

1 tblspn chopped Italian parsley

1 Heat the oil in a large frying pan over a moderate heat, add the chicken pieces and cook for 3 minutes, stirring constantly. Remove chicken and keep warm in a low oven.

2 Add the butter to the pan, then add the leeks, mushrooms, sun-dried tomatoes, red wine vinegar, lime juice, chilli, basil and parsley, cook for 3 minutes.

3 Return the chicken pieces to the frying pan, toss well. Serve immediately and garnish with fresh basil.

Serves 4

Rosemary Roasted Chicken with Carrots

900 kilojoules/215 calories per serving

4 chicken breast halves, 110g (3½ oz) each

salt

pepper

1 tblspn chopped fresh rosemary

8 carrots, cut diagonally into 5cm (2in) lengths

1 tblspn unsalted butter, cut into small cubes

2 tblspn degreased chicken stock, warmed

rosemary sprigs for garnish

1 Rub chicken with salt and freshly ground pepper to taste, sprinkle with rosemary, place in a baking dish.

Top: Chicken Pieces with Mushrooms and Basil.
Right: Lemon Honey Chicken Kebabs with Yoghurt Sauce

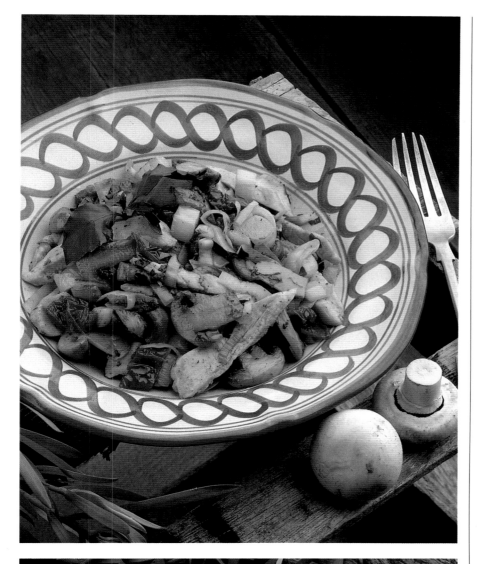

2 Boil, steam or microwave carrots until just tender, but still crisp, arrange around chicken. Dot with butter cubes.

3 Drizzle chicken with stock, bake in a 200°C (400°F) oven until cooked through, about 15 minutes.

4 Arrange chicken onto heated plates, pour over pan juices. Serve immediately, garnished with rosemary.

Serves 4

Lemon Honey Chicken Kebabs with Yoghurt Sauce

1256 kilojoules/300 calories per serving

1 tblspn butter

2 tblspn honey

3 tblspn freshly squeezed lemon juice

2 tspn apricot jam

2 tspn grated lemon rind

¼ tspn cracked black pepper

4 chicken breast fillets, cut into 2cm (¾in) cubes

2 red capsicum (pepper), cut into 2cm (¾in) pieces

½ cup low fat natural yoghurt

1 tblspn freshly squeezed lemon juice, extra

1 clove garlic, crushed

¼ tspn ground coriander

¼ tspn ground cumin

coriander sprigs for garnish

1 Melt the butter in a medium frying pan over moderate heat, add the honey, lemon juice, apricot jam, lemon rind and cracked pepper.

2 Thread the chicken pieces and capsicum pieces alternately on the skewers and place kebabs in frying pan. Cook for 1-2 minutes on all sides or until chicken is cooked through.

3 To make the sauce: Combine the yoghurt with the lemon juice, garlic, coriander and cumin.

4 Serve kebabs on a bed of saffron rice, pour sauce over the kebabs and garnish with fresh coriander.

Serves 4

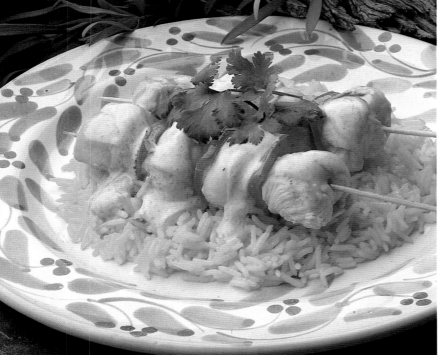

Chicken Scallopini with Raspberry Coulis

1214 kilojoules/290 calories per serving

4 single chicken breast fillets

2 eggs, lightly beaten

1 cup dried breadcrumbs

1 cup fresh raspberries

2 tspn raspberry jam

2 tblspn freshly squeezed lime juice

2 tblspn freshly squeezed orange juice

1 Dip chicken fillets in the beaten egg, then dip the chicken in breadcrumbs, shake off any excess breadcrumbs. Bake coated chicken fillets in a moderate oven for 15-20 minutes or until cooked through.

2 Meanwhile, place raspberries, jam, lime juice and orange juice in a blender or food processor, process until smooth.

3 Push pureed mixture through a sieve to catch the seeds, heat sauce in a small saucepan over low heat and serve with chicken fillets and fresh vegetables.

Serves 4

Normandy Chicken

1250 kilojoules/300 calories per serving

1 tblspn ghee

1 tblspn peanut oil

4 skinless, boneless chicken breast halves, 125g (4oz) each

salt

pepper

½ cup calvados (see note)

3 tblspn cider vinegar

500g (1lb) Jonathan apples, not peeled, cored, cut into eighths

1 cup degreased chicken stock

1 In a large frying pan heat ghee and oil, add chicken, saute over high heat until golden, about 8 minutes, turning once. Remove from pan, season to taste with salt and freshly ground pepper.

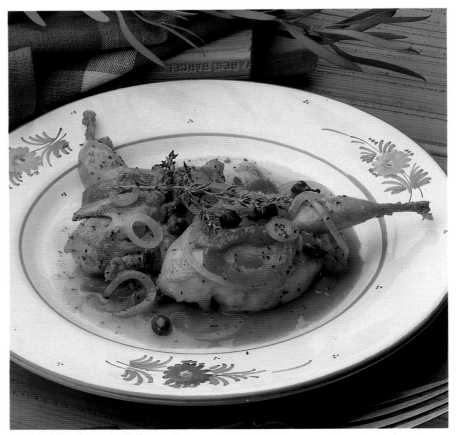

Quail with Caper Dill Sauce

2 Pour off all fat from frying pan, add half the calvados and all the vinegar. Bring to a boil, scraping up any browned bits from the bottom. Remove from the heat.

3 Place apples in a casserole, arrange chicken on top. Pour liquid in the frying pan over chicken, bake in a 180°C (350°F) oven until chicken is cooked through, about 20 minutes.

4 Remove chicken from casserole, keep warm. Pour apples and juices from pan into a processor, puree.

5 Pour in a saucepan, add stock and remaining calvados. Bring to a boil, cook until sauce thickens, about 5 minutes. Check seasoning, divide sauce among 4 heated plates, arrange chicken on top. Serve immediately.

Note: Calvados is a French apple brandy. If not available, use ordinary brandy.

Serves 4

Tarragon Chicken

837 kilojoules/200 calories per serving

2 whole chicken breasts, skin on, about 500g (1lb) each

1 large clove garlic, halved

1 lemon, halved

1 tspn dried French tarragon, chopped

salt

1 Rub chicken breasts on both sides with cut garlic and halved lemon. Very gently loosen the skin from the breast, spread tarragon between flesh and skin.

2 Place chicken on a rack in a roasting dish, squeeze over some juice of the lemon, season to taste with salt.

3 Bake in a 230°C (450°F) oven until chicken is just tender, about 35 minutes. Allow to stand at room temperature for 10 minutes.

4 Remove skin, slice meat off the bone in a single piece from each side of the breast. Serve hot.

Serves 4

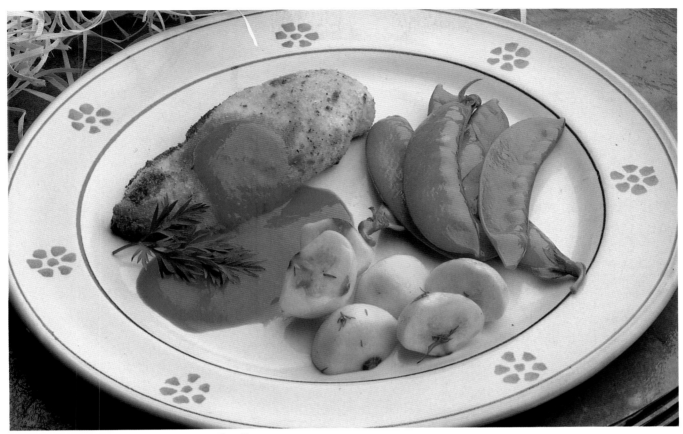

Chicken Scallopini with Raspberry Coulis

Quail with Caper Dill Sauce

1361 kilojoules/325 calories per serving

1 tblspn butter

1 onion, sliced

1 clove garlic, crushed

2 pimentos, cut into thin strips

1 tblspn honey

2 tblspn red wine vinegar

4 quails, cut in half lengthwise

1 cup dry white wine

2 tspn Dijon mustard

1 tblspn chopped fresh dill

½ tspn cracked black pepper

10 capers

fresh thyme sprigs, to garnish

1 In a large frying pan melt the butter over moderate heat. Add the onion, garlic and pimento strips, cook for 2 minutes.

2 Add the honey, wine vinegar and quails. Cook quails for 3 minutes each side.

3 Add wine, mustard, dill, black pepper and capers to the frying pan, cook until sauce thickens slightly and quails are cooked through.

4 Arrange 2 quail halves on each plate, spoon sauce over the top and garnish with fresh thyme.

Serves 4

Chicken in Red Wine

1193 kilojoules/285 calories per serving

750g (1½lb) skinless, boneless chicken breast halves

1 tblspn olive oil

1 tblspn honey

MARINADE

1½ cups dry red wine

1 tblspn olive oil

8 cloves garlic, crushed

2 tspn chopped fresh rosemary

salt

pepper

1 To make marinade: Combine wine, oil, garlic and rosemary in a large bowl, season to taste with salt and freshly ground pepper. Add chicken, cover, allow to stand at room temperature for at least 1 hour.

2 Remove chicken from marinade, pat dry with paper towels. Reserve marinade.

3 Heat oil in a non-stick frying pan, add chicken, cook until tender and golden on both sides, about 8 minutes, turning once. Place on a heated serving dish, keep warm.

4 Pour off any remaining fat from the pan, add marinade and honey, bring to a boil, scraping up any browned bits from the bottom. Cook until sauce thickens slightly.

5 Pour sauce over chicken, serve immediately.

Serves 4

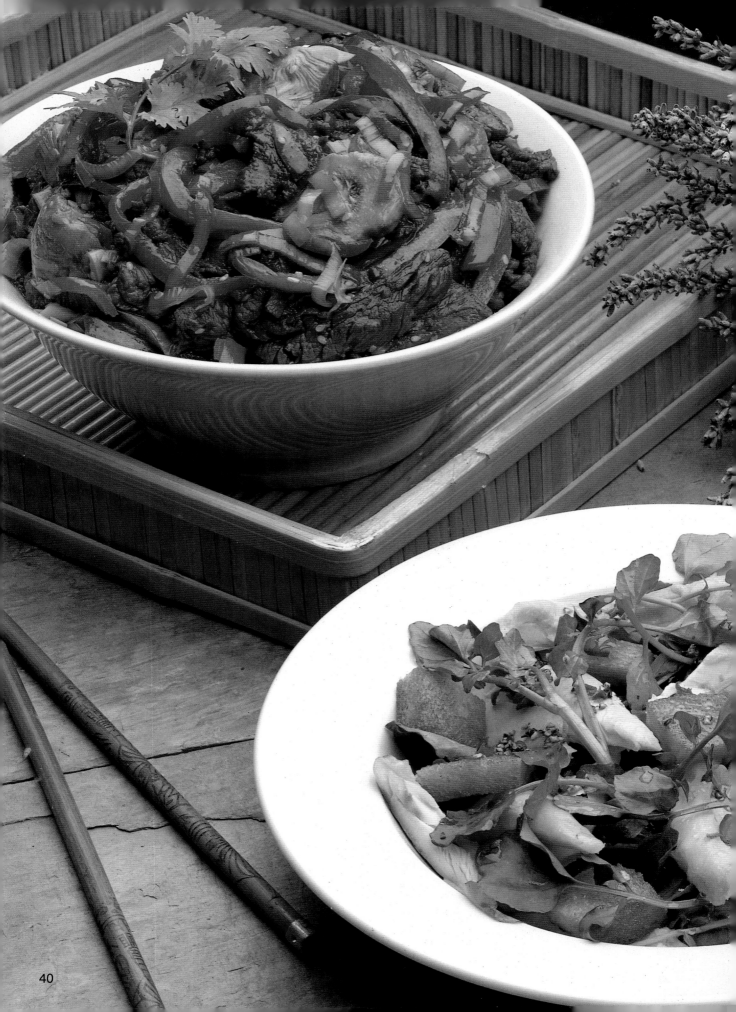

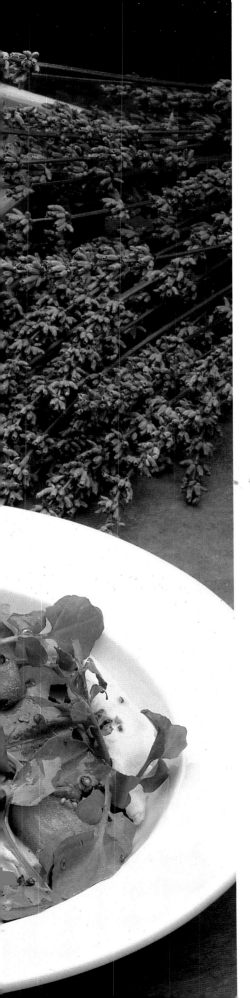

MAIN COURSE SALADS

Salads are ideal for slimmers but they need not be dull and tasteless. Try these delightful salads, you'll find them tasty and satisfying.

Oriental Beef Salad

1256 kilojoules/300 calories per serving

2 tspn oil

1 red capsium (pepper), seeded, cut into thin strips

1 green capsicum (pepper), seeded, cut into thin strips

2 leeks, trimmed and finely chopped

1 tblspn oil, extra

1 tblspn honey

2 tblspn soy sauce

625g (1lb 4oz) beef eye fillet, cut into strips

1 tspn sesame seeds

1 Heat the oil in a large frying pan, over medium heat. Add the red and green capsicum and the leeks and fry for 2 minutes. Remove with a slotted spoon and set aside.

2 Add the extra oil, honey and soy sauce to the frying pan and heat.

3 Add the beef and cook for 3 minutes, or until cooked through, stirring constantly.

4 Stir in sesame seeds and reserved vegetables, serve immediately.

Serves 4

Smoked Chicken and Watercress Salad with Croutons

963 kilojoules/230 calories per serving

1½ tblspn lite margarine

2 cloves garlic, crushed

4 slices bread, crusts removed

2 cups watercress sprigs

1½ cups smoked chicken, torn into bite-size pieces

2 tblspn low-joule French dressing

1 Melt the margarine in a small frying pan over moderate heat. Add the garlic and cook for 1 minute.

2 Cut each slice of bread into 9 squares and add to the frying pan. Cook on both sides until light golden brown, drain on absorbent paper.

3 Arrange the watercress and chicken pieces on a serving plate. Pour over French dressing and toss gently.

4 Arrange croutons on top and serve immediately.

Serves 4

Top: Oriental Beef Salad. Bottom: Smoked Chicken and Watercress Salad with Croutons

Deep Sea Perch Salad

1884 kilojoules/450 calories per serving

1kg (2lb) deep sea perch (sea bass, catfish) fillets

500g (1lb) very thin fettucine

2 zucchini (courgette), julienned

2 carrots, julienned

2 stalks celery, julienned

4 leeks, thoroughly rinsed, julienned

MARINADE

juice of 2 lemons

2 tblspn chopped fresh parsley

pinch of cayenne pepper

salt

pepper

DRESSING

1 tspn Dijon mustard

2 tblspn chopped fresh dill

2 tblspn freshly squeezed lemon juice

4 tblspn safflower oil

1 To make marinade: Combine lemon juice, parsley and cayenne pepper in a screwtop jar, season to taste with salt and freshly ground pepper. Shake well to blend.

2 Cut fish fillets into bite-size pieces. Pour over marinade, cover, stand at room temperature for 40 minutes.

3 To make the dressing: In a bowl mix together mustard, dill, salt and pepper to taste, and lemon juice. Gradually add oil, whisking continuously, until dressing is thoroughly amalgamated.

4 Cook pasta in boiling salted water for 3 minutes if fresh, or 8-10 minutes if dried. Drain, rinse under cold water and place in a large salad bowl. Toss with half the dressing.

5 Steam julienned vegetables over boiling water for 1 minute. Add fish, steam a further 1-2 minutes, or until fish is opaque. Set aside and cool.

6 Mound fettucine on a serving platter. Top with fish and vegetables. Pour over remaining dressing and serve immediately.

Serves 6

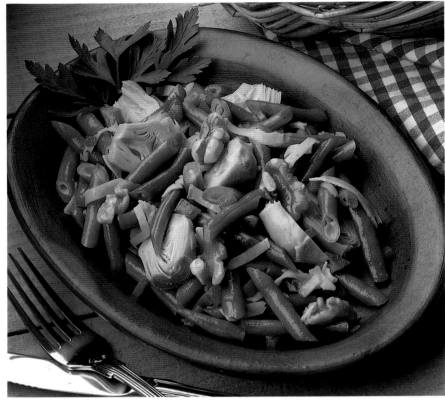
Artichoke, Ham and Fresh Bean Salad

Artichoke, Ham and Fresh Bean Salad

984 kilojoules/235 calories per serving

300g (10oz) fresh green beans

6 artichoke hearts, halved

155g (5oz) ham, finely sliced into strips

2 tblspn finely chopped red capsicum (pepper)

10 walnut pieces

2 tspn walnut oil

1 tblspn freshly squeezed lime juice

sprig of Italian parsley

1 Top and tail beans and cut into 2cm (¾in) lengths. Bring a large saucepan of water to the boil, add beans and cook for 1 minute. Remove with a slotted spoon and refresh under cold water.

2 Combine the beans with the artichoke hearts, ham, red capsicum and walnuts.

3 Arrange salad on serving plate and dress with combined walnut oil and lime juice. Garnish with fresh parsley if desired.

Serves 4

Katie's Healthy Lunch Box Salad

1026 kilojoules/245 calories per serving

4 cups lettuce, torn into bite-size pieces

1 cup chopped tomatoes

1 cup chopped celery

1 cup chopped cucumber

125g (4oz) low fat Cheddar cheese, grated

1 carrot, grated

2 tblspn finely chopped chives

2½ tblspn freshly squeezed lemon juice

DRESSING

2 cups chopped cooked asparagus

4 tblspn plain low fat yoghurt

½ tspn garlic powder

salt

pepper

2 tblspn chopped fresh dill

2 hard-boiled eggs, quartered

1 Combine lettuce, tomato, celery, cucumber, cheese, carrot and chives. Sprinkle with half the lemon juice. Toss well and chill.

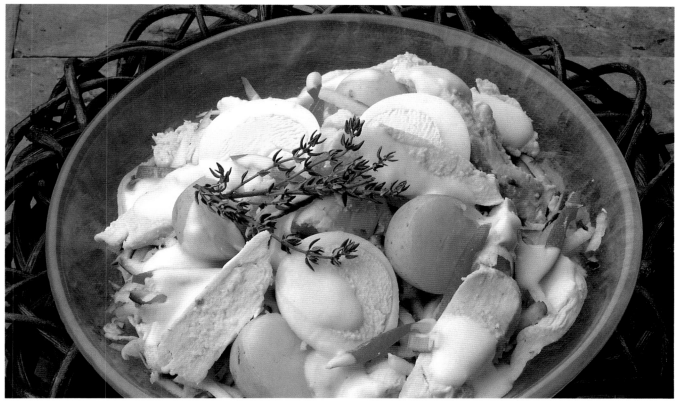

Chicken Potato Salad with Thyme and Mayonnaise

2 To make dressing: In a bowl, blend together asparagus, yoghurt and garlic, season to taste with salt, freshly ground pepper and the remaining lemon juice, if desired.

3 Spoon dressing over chilled salad and garnish with dill and hard-boiled eggs.

Serves 4

Chicken Potato Salad with Thyme and Mayonnaise

1214 kilojoules/290 calories per serving

2 cups cooked chicken, skin removed, cut into bite-size pieces

4 zucchini (courgettes), grated

1 tspn chopped fresh thyme

8 baby potatoes, boiled and halved

1 red capsicum (pepper), seeded and sliced into thin strips

4 hard-boiled eggs, peeled and sliced

1 tblspn chopped fresh coriander

¼ cup low-joule French dressing

2 tblspn low-joule mayonnaise

1 In a medium bowl, combine chicken, zucchini, thyme and potatoes; mix well.

2 Arrange chicken mixture on serving plate, top with the red capsicum strips, coriander and egg slices.

3 Pour over combined dressing and mayonnaise and serve chilled.

Serves 4

Light Summer Salad with Tomato Dressing

775 kilojoules/185 calories per serving

2 Spanish onions

2 green capsicum (pepper), seeded

125g (4oz) fennel

250g (½lb) zucchini (courgette)

8 tomatoes

1 stalk celery

2 avocados

sprig of oregano for garnish

TOMATO DRESSING

4 tomatoes, peeled and chopped

2 tblspn tomato puree

juice of 1 lemon

2 tblspn olive oil

1 tspn chopped fresh oregano

1 tspn chopped fresh thyme

2 cloves garlic, finely chopped

1 To make Tomato Dressing: Combine tomatoes, tomato puree and lemon juice in a bowl. Gradually whisk in oil, herbs and garlic. Cover, stand at room temperature for 1 hour.

2 Slice onions, capsicums and fennel into very thin rings. Place in a salad bowl. Finely slice zucchini, tomato, celery and avocado. Add to vegetables in salad bowl.

3 Pour over dressing and garnish with a sprig of oregano.

Serves 8

43

Beef and Black Bean Salad

1758 kilojoules/420 calories per serving

315g (10oz) black kidney beans, soaked overnight

1 onion, chopped

2 cloves garlic, finely chopped

2 tspn chopped fresh thyme

pinch of cayenne pepper

1 bay leaf

1 tblspn olive oil

2 leeks, washed thoroughly, thinly sliced

750g (1½lb) fillet steak, trimmed of all fat and sliced into thin strips

250g (½lb) French beans, trimmed, cut in half

1 onion, extra

8 cherry tomatoes, halved

1 green capsicum (pepper), seeded, cut into strips

1 butter lettuce

DRESSING

¾ cup red wine vinegar

juice of 1 lemon

2 tblspn Dijon mustard

2 tblspn honey

salt

pepper

2 cloves garlic, finely chopped

¼ cup safflower oil

4 tblspn virgin olive oil

1 Drain beans, place in a large casserole with onion, garlic, thyme, cayenne pepper and bay leaf. Cover with cold water, bring to a boil. Reduce heat to a simmer, cover casserole, cook for 1½ hours or until beans are just tender. Drain, rinse beans under cold running water. Set aside.

2 Heat oil in a non-stick frying pan, add leeks and cook for 2-3 minutes. Add beef strips and saute 2 minutes. Set aside.

3 Cook French beans in boiling salted water for 3-4 minutes. Drain and refresh under cold running water.

4 To make dressing: Combine all ingredients, except the oils, in a processor. Process for 15 seconds. Gradually add oils, process until well amalgamated.

5 In a large bowl combine onion, tomato, green capsicum and beef. Add black beans and French beans, pour over half the salad dressing, toss well to coat. Make a bed of lettuce leaves on a large platter, arrange salad mixture on top. Serve immediately, with remaining dressing separately.

Serves 8-10

Tossed Mediterranean Salad

670 kilojoules/160 calories per serving

1 endive or coral lettuce

10 stuffed green olives, halved

5 black olives, pitted and sliced

4 hard-boiled eggs, peeled and sliced

1 red capsicum (pepper), seeded and cut into thin strips

2 celery stalks, cut into thin strips

2 tblspn red wine vinegar

1 tspn honey

1 tblspn freshly squeezed lime juice

1 tspn olive oil

1 Wash lettuce and break into pieces. Arrange lettuce, green olives, black olives, sliced eggs, red capsicum and celery strips on salad plate.

2 Mix together the wine vinegar, honey, lime juice and oil and pour over salad.

Serves 4

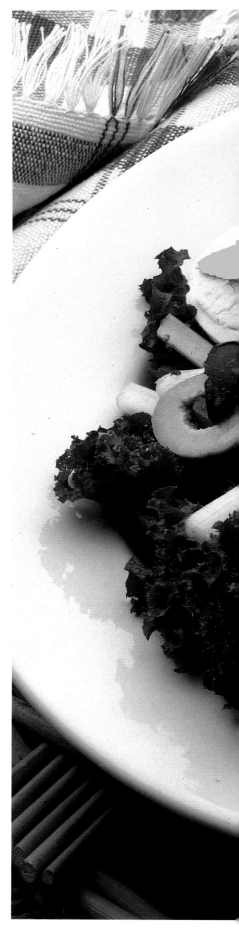

Tossed Mediterranean Salad

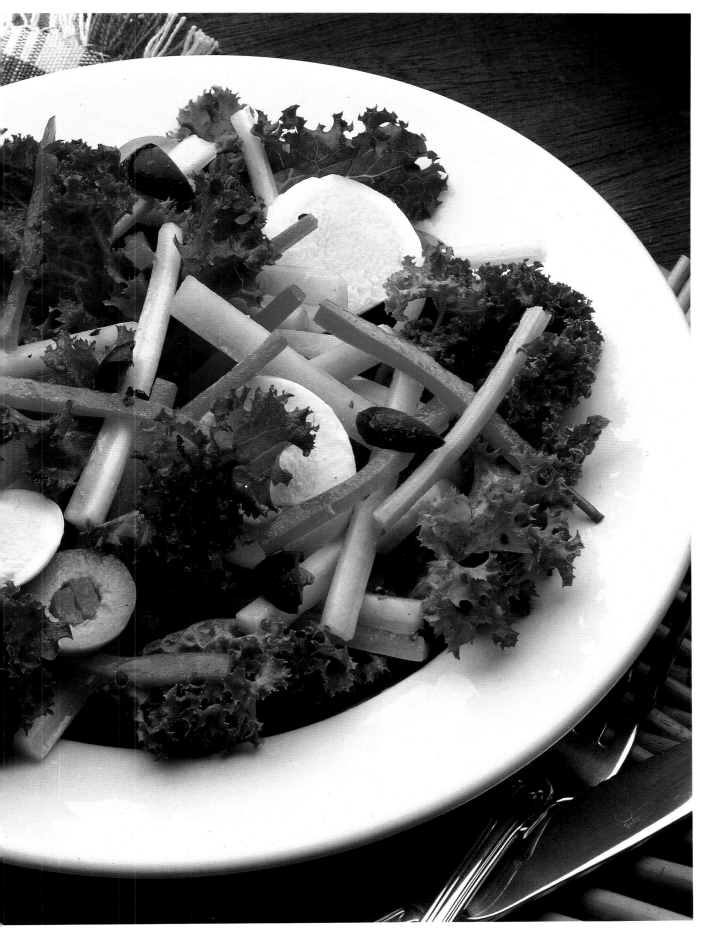

Salmon Toasties and Avocado

1633 kilojoules/390 calories per serving

2 x 210g (7oz) cans salmon, drained, bones removed

4 spring onions (scallions), chopped

2 tblspn chopped fresh parsley

½ red capsicum (pepper), seeded and finely chopped

½ tspn cracked black pepper

1 tblspn freshly squeezed lemon juice

8 slices bread, crusts removed and toasted

8 coral lettuce leaves

1 lime, sliced

1 avocado, peeled, seeded and sliced

1 Combine salmon, spring onions, parsley, red capsicum, pepper and lemon juice in a medium bowl.

2 Arrange salmon and toasts on serving plate, garnish with lettuce, lime slices and avocado.

Serves 4

Turkey Breast and Feta Salad

2072 kilojoules/495 calories per serving

1kg (2lb) cooked turkey breast, skin removed, cut into bite-size pieces

2 stalks celery, finely chopped

2 cucumbers, peeled, halved, seeded

12 large black olives, stoned, halved

250g (½lb) feta cheese, cubed

1 bunch curly endive

1 small bunch watercress

VINAIGRETTE

3 cloves garlic, finely chopped

4 tblspn chopped fresh basil

1 tspn sugar

2 tblspn whole grain mustard

freshly ground pepper to taste

4 tblspn freshly squeezed lemon juice

4 tblspn red wine vinegar

4 tblspn safflower oil

8 tblspn virgin olive oil

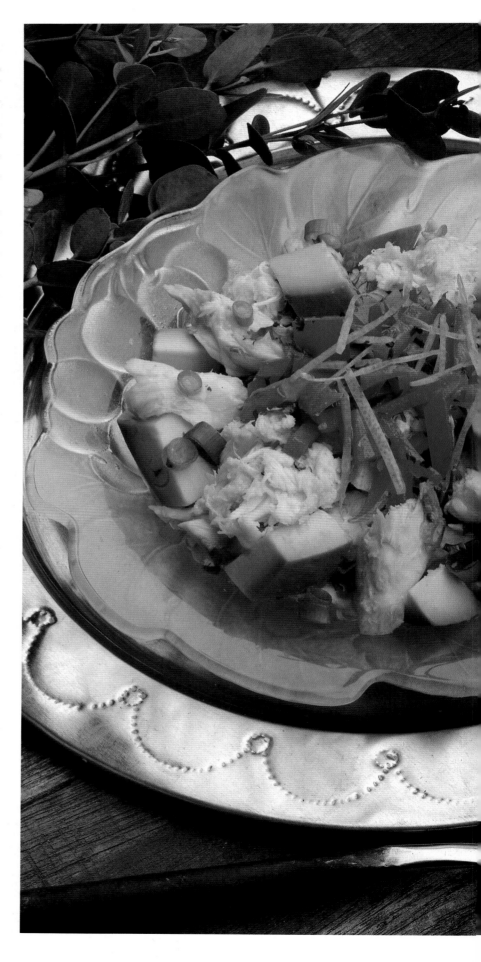

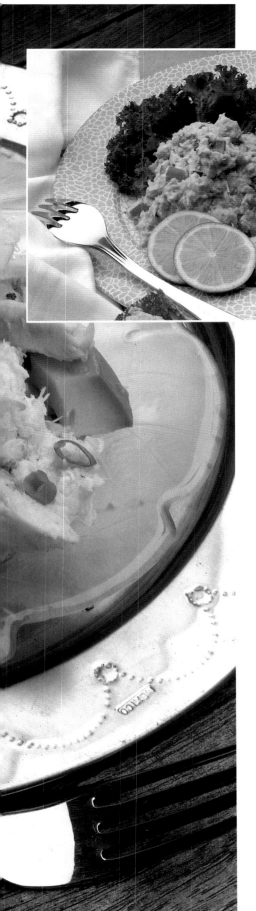

Left: Crab and Gemfish Salad with Avocado. Below: Salmon Toasties with Avocado

1 To make vinaigrette: Combine all ingredients in a screwtop jar, shake until well blended.

2 Combine turkey, celery, cucumber, olives and cheese in a bowl. Pour over dressing, toss well to coat.

3 Arrange endive leaves on individual plates. Spoon salad on top and garnish with watercress leaves. Serve immediately.

Serves 8

Crab and Gemfish Salad with Avocado

879 kilojoules/210 calories per serving

4 crabs, cooked

½ cup dry white wine

2 tblspn freshly squeezed lime juice

400g (13oz) gemfish (sea bream, orange roughy) fillets, skin removed

1 tblspn finely chopped spring onions (scallions)

¼ tspn cracked black pepper

2 tblspn freshly squeezed lemon juice

1 medium avocado, peeled, pitted and cut into large pieces

1 tspn finely chopped coriander

¼ red capsicum (pepper), seeded and chopped

orange or lemon rind for garnish, cut into thin strips

1 Remove the flesh from the crab shells and set aside.

2 In a large deep frying pan, heat the wine and lime juice over moderate heat until boiling. Reduce heat, simmer.

3 Add the gemfish fillets and cook until opaque. Remove with a slotted spoon and set aside to cool.

4 Flake the fish and combine with the crab, spring onions, pepper, lemon juice and avocado.

5 Sprinkle chopped coriander and red capsicum over the top and garnish with strips of rind.

Serves 4

Chicken Salad with Mango and Spanish Onion Dressing

775 kilojoules/185 calories per serving

500g (1lb) chicken breasts, skin on

1 mango, peeled, stoned, flesh coarsely chopped

juice of ½ a lemon

1 tblspn red wine vinegar

1 tblspn olive oil

salt

pepper

radicchio leaves

½ small Spanish onion, chopped

1 Place chicken breasts under a pre-heated griller, cook about 8 minutes, turning once, or until chicken is tender. Set aside to cool.

2 Combine mango flesh, lemon juice, vinegar and oil in a processor. Puree until smooth, season to taste with salt and freshly ground pepper.

3 Arrange radicchio leaves on a platter.

4 When chicken is cool, remove all skin, cut flesh into strips. Arrange on radicchio leaves.

5 Stir onion into mango mixture, pour mixture over chicken. Cover salad and refrigerate for 30 minutes before serving.

Serves 6

10 MOST COMMON REASONS WHY DIETS DON'T WORK

1 Fad diets — eg the grapefruit diet. The only way to diet successfully is to eat a balanced diet, with all the basic five food groups represented. The groups are:
a) milk and cheese
b) bread and cereal
c) vegetables and fruits
d) meat, poultry, fish, nuts and dried beans
e) fats, sweets and alcohol

2 Expecting too rapid a weight loss — generally speaking, weight which is lost slowly but steadily will stay off. When weight is lost too rapidly, the diet is often too difficult to sustain and lacking in necessary nutrients. Do not weigh yourself every day, once a week is sufficient.

3 Taking pills to lose weight — definitely a no-no. With a sensible diet and regular exercise everyone should be able to lose weight.

4 Giving up food you really like — this is a very unwise move. The more you ban favourite foods from your diet, the more you will crave them. Allow yourself a little treat every now and then, eg have 1 chocolate biscuit, but don't eat the whole packet!

5 Not eating three meals a day — by skipping breakfast and even lunch, some people think they will cut kilojoules. They are only kidding themselves. By dinnertime they are usually so hungry, they could eat the proverbial horse, and some do!

6 Not exercising — you cannot lose weight and keep it off by dieting alone. Regular exercise is the cornerstone of any solid weight loss programme, even if the exercise is simply walking instead of driving, walking the stairs rather than riding the lift. And by the way, the best exercise of all: place your hands very firmly on the edge of the table and push your chair backwards.

7 Choosing a diet plan that is not right for you — maybe your friend had spectacular results with a particular diet; this does not mean it will work for you. Choose a diet which fits in with your lifestyle, or you'll never be able to sustain it.

8 Losing weight for the wrong reasons — the only way your weight will come off and stay off, is when you're motivated from within to follow a sensible diet plan; not when you try to lose weight because your man would like you better slim, or your sister says you could look more like her if only you...

9 By Christmas/my wedding day/the ball I want to lose 6 kilos — this may work, but what after Christmas/your wedding day or the ball? You'll put on weight again unless you follow a sensible diet plan.

10 I ate a lot of chickpeas, because I read somewhere it's good for me — yes, chickpeas are very good for you, but they are also very calorific. Dried beans play a very important part in a balanced diet, but keep watching the kilojoules!

EIGHT SUPER MENUS

SUMMER LUNCH

Cold Cucumber and Dill Soup

Watercress and Fennel Salad

Salmon Frittata

Sparkling Strawberries

With these delicious complete meals, you can plan special occasions and still know that you're within your slimming dietary guidelines.

MEDITERRANEAN DINNER

Pimento and Tomato Soup

Eggplant (Aubergine) and Mint Bake

Poached Tuna with Rosemary on Blanched Asparagus

Fresh Berry Compote in Yoghurt Brandy Sauce

WINTER LUNCH

Individual Pizzas

Chicken Potentina

Brussel Sprouts and Almonds

Champagne Zabaglione with Oranges

ORIENTAL DINNER

Crab Soup

Cellophane Noodle Salad

Beef and Vegetable Stir-Fry

Oriental Oranges with Yoghurt

VEGETARIAN LUNCH

Fennel and Orange Salad with Orange Vinaigrette

Cheesy Rice Ring with Garlic Vegetables

Spicy Bean and Vegetable Salad

Lemon and Basil Granita

SPRING DINNER

Endive and Snowpea Salad

Pasta Primavera with Tomato Basil Sauce

Scallops with Julienne Vegetables and Tomato Coulis

Three Fruit Compote

WINTER DINNER

Fresh Parmesan Cheese Salad with Croutons

Bacon and Bean Casserole with Barley

Red Cabbage with Caraway Seeds

Tangy Pear and Raspberry Cobbler

CELEBRATION DINNER

Mussels in Wine and Tomato Sauce

Chicken Breasts with Green Sauce

Spicy Baked Potatoes

Fluffy Blueberry Mousse

SUMMER LUNCH

Cold Cucumber and Dill Soup

Watercress and Fennel Salad

Salmon Frittata

Sparkling Strawberries

Watercress and Fennel Salad

209 kilojoules/50 calories per serving

4 cups watercress

1 small fennel bulb, halved and sliced into small pieces

8 walnut pieces

2 tblspn lite French dressing

2 tspn olive oil

1 clove garlic, crushed

1 Arrange watercress, fennel and walnuts on a serving plate.

2 Pour combined French dressing, olive oil and garlic over salad, serve immediately.

Serves 4

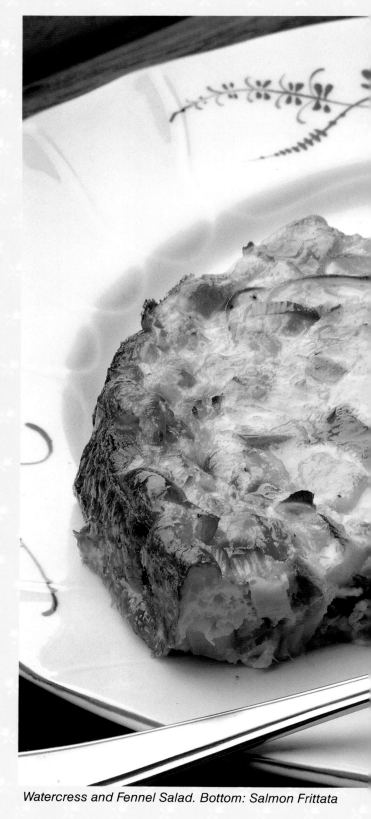

Watercress and Fennel Salad. Bottom: Salmon Frittata

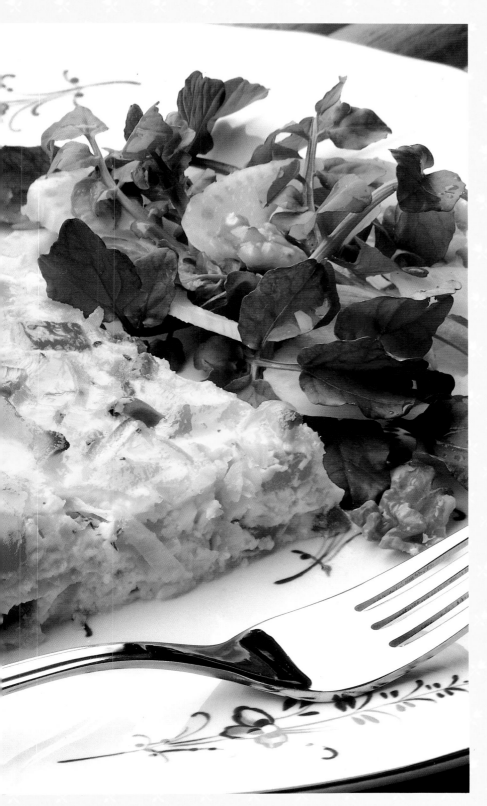

Salmon Frittata

607 kilojoules/145 calories per serving

1 tblspn lite margarine

1 onion, chopped

2 spring onions (scallions), finely chopped

½ green capsicum (pepper), seeded, finely chopped

1 leek, finely sliced, white part only

1 tomato, chopped

155g (5oz) smoked salmon, chopped

4 eggs

¾ cup skim milk

½ tspn cracked black pepper

1 Melt the margarine in a medium frying pan, add the onion, spring onions, capsicum and leeks, cook for 4 minutes.

2 Add the tomato and salmon, cook for 1 minute, remove from heat. Cool mixture to room temperature.

3 Beat the eggs with the milk, add the pepper and stir the mixture into the cooled vegetable salmon mixture.

4 Pour mixture into a greased ovenproof 20cm (8in) flan dish and bake in a moderate oven for 25 minutes.

Serves 6

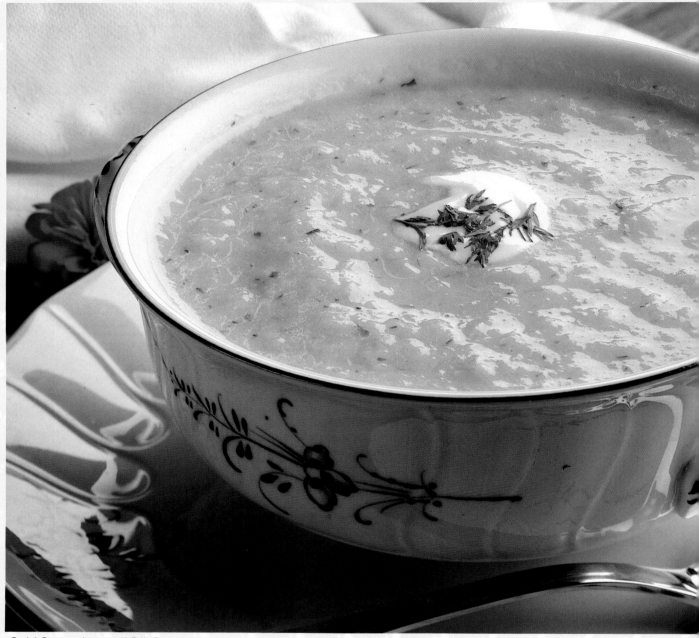

Cold Cucumber and Dill Soup

Cold Cucumber and Dill Soup

314 kilojoules/75 calories per serving

4 cups degreased chicken stock

1 large onion, finely chopped

1 leek, finely chopped, white part only

2 tblspn chopped fresh dill

2 cucumbers, peeled, seeded and chopped

1 potato, peeled and chopped

¼ cup natural yoghurt

1 tblspn chopped fresh dill, extra

1 Bring stock to the boil in a large saucepan, add the onion, leeks, dill, cucumbers and potato, cook for 20 minutes or until potato is tender.

2 Remove vegetables with a slotted spoon and reserve 1 cup of the stock, discarding remaining stock. Puree vegetables and the 1 cup stock in a food processor or blender until smooth.

3 Chill soup for several hours, serve cold with a teaspoon of yoghurt on top, sprinkle extra dill on yoghurt.

Serves 4

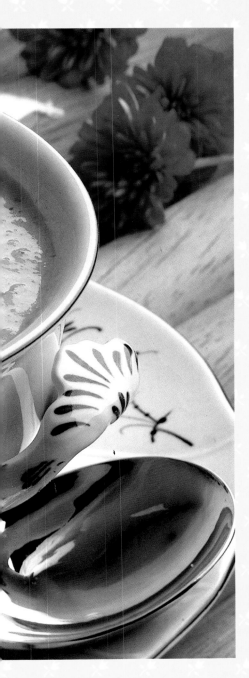

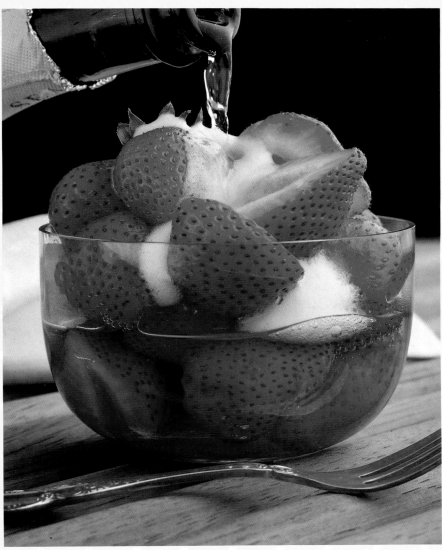

Sparkling Strawberries

Sparkling Strawberries

921 kilojoules/220 calories per serving

4 cups large strawberries, hulled and halved

2 cups champagne

¼ cup Cointreau

1 Marinate the strawberries in 1 cup of champagne and the Cointreau for 2 hours.

2 Divide strawberries between each serving glass, pour the remaining champagne over the strawberries, serve immediately.

Serves 4

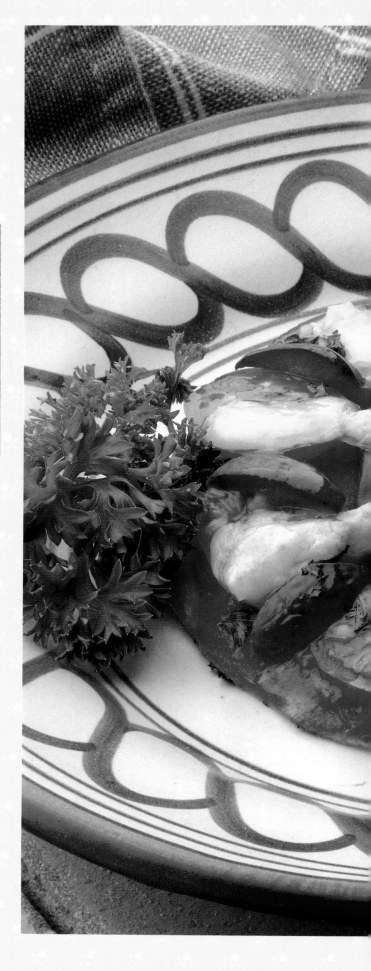

WINTER LUNCH

Individual Pizzas

Chicken Potentina

Brussel Sprouts and Almonds

*Champagne Zabaglione
with Oranges*

Individual Pizzas

879 kilojoules/210 calories per serving

4 small wholemeal pocket breads

2 tblspn tomato paste

½ cup sliced cherry tomatoes

¼ cup black olives, pitted and cut into small strips

100g (3½oz) mozzarella cheese, cut into thin strips

2 tspn finely chopped parsley

1 Trim each pocket bread to make 4 small rounds of bread, about 10-12cm (4-5in) diameter. Toast one side of the bread rounds.

2 Spread the untoasted side with tomato paste, arrange tomato slices, olive strips and cheese in a wheel shape on top of the tomato paste.

3 Sprinkle parsley on top and bake in a moderate oven for about 7 minutes or until cheese has melted. Serve immediately.

Serves 4

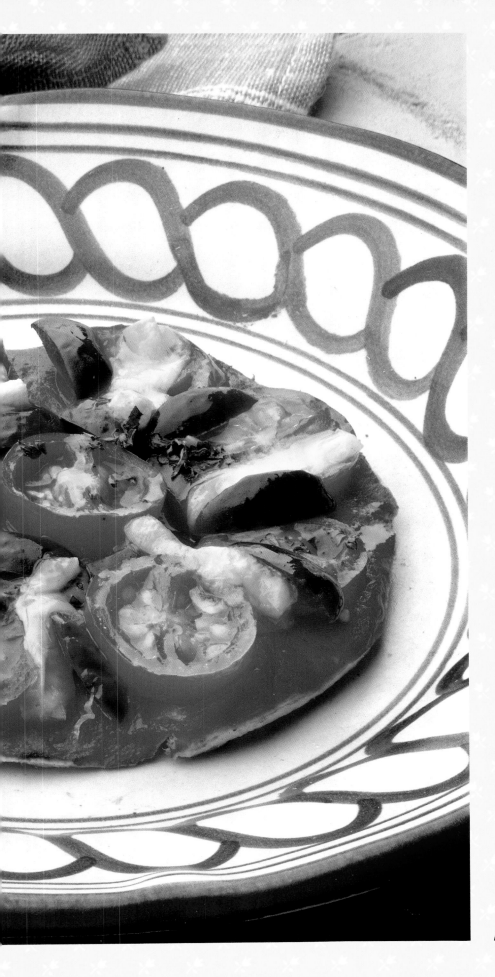

Individual Pizzas

Chicken Potentina

1068 kilojoules/255 calories per serving

1 tblspn lite margarine

1 onion, peeled and chopped

6 slices prosciutto, cut into strips

4 chicken breast fillets

½ cup dry white wine

425g (13½oz) can Italian peeled tomatoes and juice

1 tblspn chopped basil

1 tblspn chopped parsley

1 Melt the margarine over moderate heat in a large frying pan. Add the onion and prosciutto, cook for 4 minutes. Add the chicken fillets and cook for 3 minutes each side.

2 Add half the wine and cook until wine evaporates. Add the remaining ¼ cup of wine, tomatoes and their juice, basil and parsley. Cook mixture for a further 10-15 minutes or until chicken is tender.

3 Serve the chicken fillets on a small platter, top with the tomato-wine sauce and serve immediately. Garnish with a fresh basil sprig if desired.

Serves 4

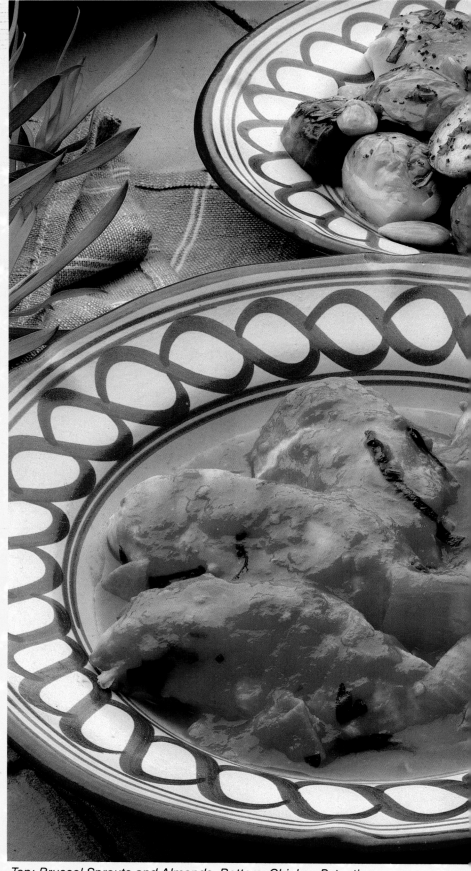

*Top: Brussel Sprouts and Almonds. Bottom: Chicken Potentina.
Above Right: Champagne Zabaglione with Oranges*

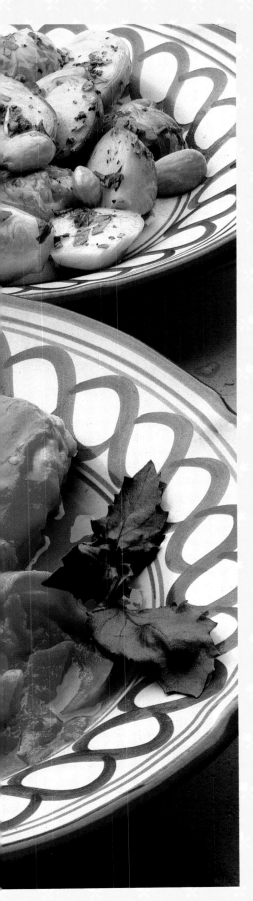

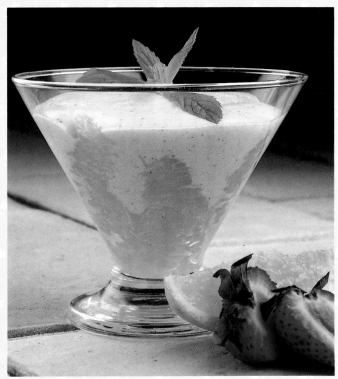

Brussel Sprouts and Almonds

314 kilojoules/75 calories per serving

400g (13oz) brussel sprouts, cut in halves

¼ cup blanched almonds, toasted

¼ tspn cracked black pepper

¼ tspn sambal oelek (chilli paste)

1 tspn finely chopped mint

2 tblspn freshly squeezed lime juice

1 tblspn olive oil

1 Bring a large saucepan of water to the boil, add the brussel sprouts and cook for 4 minutes or until just cooked. Drain and refresh under cold water, drain.

2 Arrange brussel sprouts and almonds on a serving plate. Dress with combined black pepper, sambal oelek, mint, lime juice and olive oil.

Serves 4

Champagne Zabaglione with Oranges

712 kilojoules/170 calories per serving

2 large navel oranges, peeled and segmented

3 large egg yolks

2 tblspn sugar

¼ tspn cinnamon

½ cup champagne

1 Drain the orange segments in a strainer.

2 Place the egg yolks, sugar and cinnamon in the top of a double boiler saucepan. Place about 5cm (2in) of water in the bottom saucepan and place over moderate heat.

3 Whisk the eggs, sugar and cinnamon over the simmering water until pale yellow and slightly thickened.

4 Add half of the champagne and continue to whisk until foamy. Add the remaining champagne and beat for a further 5 minutes.

5 Divide the orange segments between 4 serving glasses, spoon the sauce over the oranges.

Serves 4

SPRING DINNER

Endive and Snowpea Salad

*Pasta Primavera with
Tomato Basil Sauce*

*Scallops with Julienne Vegetables
and Tomato Coulis*

Three Fruit Compote

Endive and Snowpea Salad

251 kilojoules/60 calories per serving

200g (6½oz) fresh snowpeas

1 curly endive, leaves torn into bite-size pieces

1 orange, sliced and cut into small wedges

3 tblspn freshly squeezed orange juice

2 tspn finely grated orange rind

1 tblspn freshly squeezed lime juice

1 tblspn olive oil

2 tspn finely chopped fresh parsley

¼ tspn cracked black pepper

1 Bring a medium saucepan of water to the boil, add the snowpeas and cook for 30 seconds. Remove with a slotted spoon and refresh under cold water.

2 Arrange the endive leaves, snowpeas and orange slices in salad bowl and dress with combined orange juice, orange rind, lime juice, olive oil, parsley and pepper.

Serves 4

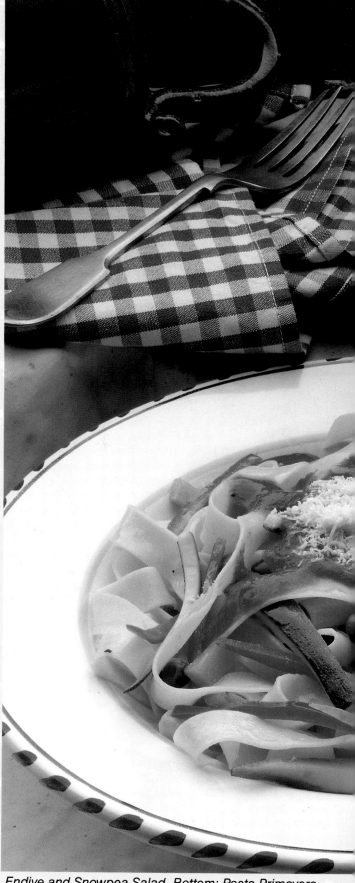

Endive and Snowpea Salad. Bottom: Pasta Primavera with Tomato Basil Sauce

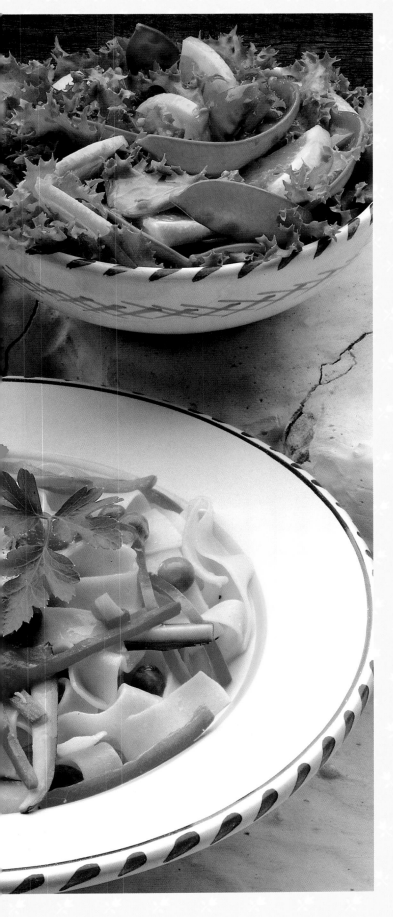

Pasta Primavera with Tomato Basil Sauce

963 kilojoules/230 calories per serving

400g (13oz) dried fettucine

½ cup frozen peas, thawed, blanched

1 red capsicum (pepper), cut into thin strips, blanched

2 zucchini (courgette), cut into thin strips, blanched

½ cup peeled pumpkin, cut into small cubes, blanched

1 tblspn olive oil

¼ tspn black pepper

3 tomatoes, chopped

1 tblspn chopped fresh basil

2 cloves garlic, crushed

2 tblspn tomato paste

4 tblspn freshly grated Parmesan cheese

1 Bring a large saucepan of water to the boil, add the fettucine and cook until just tender; drain.

2 Add the peas, red capsicum, zucchini, pumpkin, oil and pepper to the fettucine, toss well. Divide pasta between four serving plates.

3 Meanwhile, puree tomatoes, basil, garlic and tomato paste in a food processor until smooth, pour mixture through a sieve and heat in a small saucepan over moderate heat.

4 Spoon 3 tablespoons of the sauce on pasta, sprinkle 1 tablespoon of cheese on top. Serve immediately.

Serves 4

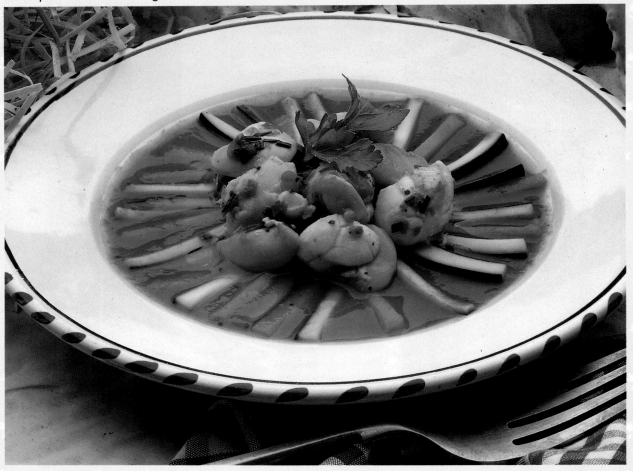

Scallops with Julienne Vegetables and Tomato Coulis

544 kilojoules/130 calories per serving

2 tblspn freshly squeezed lime juice

½ cup dry white wine

¼ cup cracked black pepper

¼ tspn sambal oelek (chilli paste)

400g (13oz) scallops, deveined

2 carrots, peeled and cut into thin strips

2 zucchini (courgette), peeled and cut into thin strips

1 large tomato, chopped

1 tblspn chopped chives

¾ cup tomato puree

1 clove garlic, crushed

1 Heat the lime juice, wine, pepper and chilli paste with ¼ cup water in a medium frying pan until simmering. Add the scallops and poach for 2 minutes, remove with a slotted spoon and set aside.

2 Bring a large saucepan of water to the boil, add the carrots and zucchini and cook for 1 minute. Remove with a slotted spoon, refresh under cold water, drain.

3 To make coulis: Place tomato, chives, puree and garlic in a blender or food processor, blend until smooth. Pour mixture through a sieve, then heat gently until hot, over moderate heat, in a small saucepan.

4 To serve, spoon 3 tablespoons of the tomato coulis onto each serving plate. Decoratively arrange vegetable strips on the coulis, place scallops on a mound on vegetables. Serve immediately.

Serves 4

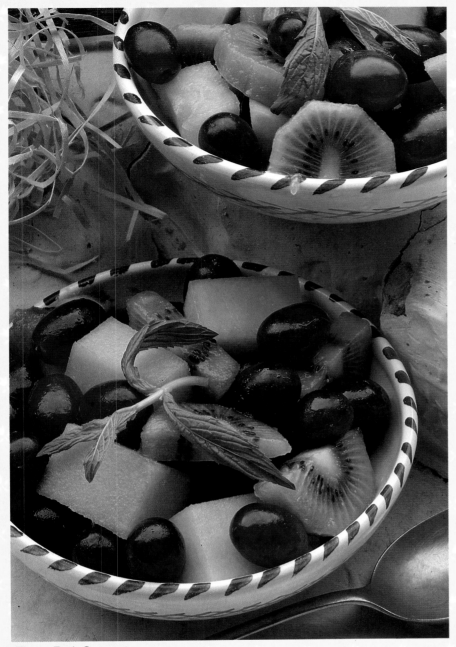

Three Fruit Compote

Three Fruit Compote

921 kilojoules/220 calories per serving

1 rockmelon (cantaloupe), peeled, seeded and cut into 2cm (¾in) cubes

2 kiwi fruit, peeled and sliced

2 cups red grapes

3 tblspn freshly squeezed lime juice

1 tblspn honey

¼ tspn ground cinnamon

mint sprigs to garnish

1 Divide the fruit between 4 serving dishes and chill.

2 Just before serving, mix together the lime juice, honey and cinnamon and pour over the fruit. Decorate with a sprig of mint if desired.

Serves 4

ORIENTAL DINNER

Crab Soup

Cellophane Noodle Salad

Beef and Vegetable Stir-Fry

Oriental Oranges with Yoghurt

Cellophane Noodle Salad

502 kilojoules/120 calories per serving

315g (10oz) cellophane noodles

1 large carrot, peeled and chopped into very small pieces

5 finely chopped spring onions (scallions)

1 tblspn sesame oil

1 tblspn white wine vinegar

2 tblspn freshly squeezed lime juice

1 Soak the noodles in hot water until softened, about 30 minutes.

2 Drain well and toss with the carrot, spring onions, oil, wine vinegar and lime juice.

Serves 4

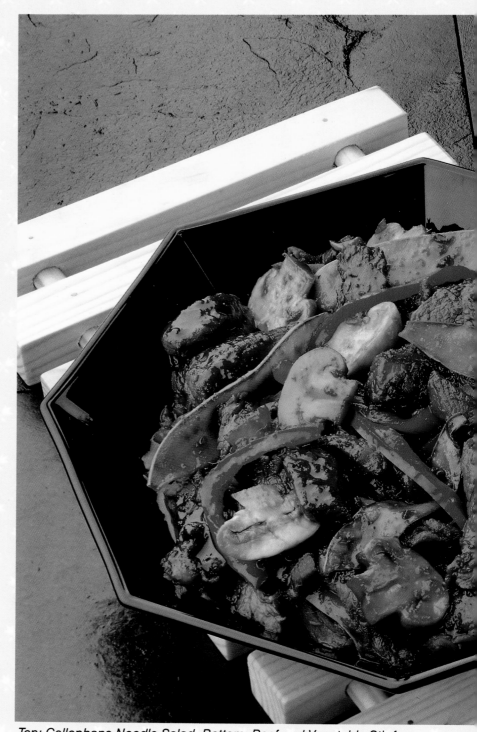

Top: Cellophane Noodle Salad. Bottom: Beef and Vegetable Stir-fry

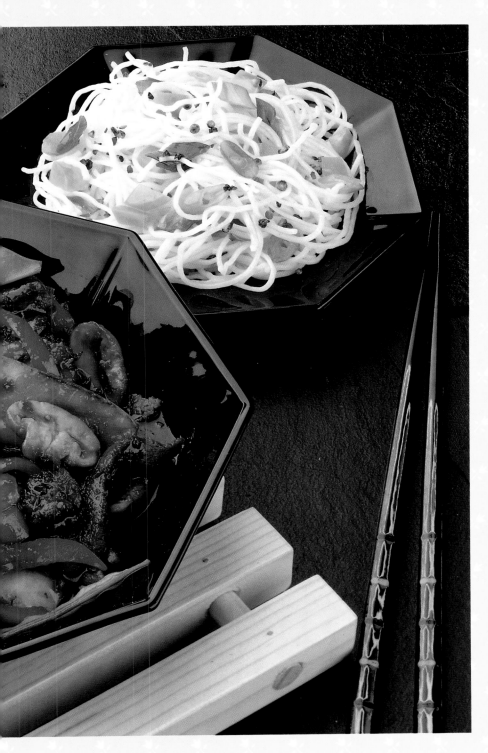

Beef and Vegetable Stir-fry

1047 kilojoules/250 calories per serving

½ cup water

¼ cup soy sauce

2 tblspn honey

2 tspn grated fresh ginger

1 tspn sesame oil

3 cloves garlic, crushed

500g (1lb) eye fillet of beef, cut into strips

1 tblspn oil

155g (5oz) button mushrooms, sliced

1 red capsicum (pepper), seeded, cut into thin strips

100g (3½oz) snowpeas, trimmed

1 In a medium bowl, combine the water, soy sauce, honey, ginger, sesame oil, garlic and sliced beef, mix well, cover, refrigerate for 2 hours.

2 Heat the oil in a large frying pan over moderate heat. Remove the beef from marinade with a slotted spoon and add to the hot frying pan, cook for 3 minutes, remove with slotted spoon and set aside. Reserve marinade.

3 Add the mushrooms and capsicum to the frying pan, cook for 3 minutes. Pour in the marinade and bring to a simmer. Boil mixture until sauce thickens slightly, about 3 minutes.

4 Stir in the meat and snowpeas, serve immediately.

Serves 4

Crab Soup

670 kilojoules/160 calories per serving

2 tspn olive oil

½ cup chopped spring onions (scallions)

1 pimento, drained and chopped

4 bacon rashers, rind and fat removed, chopped

1 cup canned chicken soup

3 cups degreased chicken stock

2 tblspn cornflour, dissolved in 3 tblspn water

1½ cups freshly cooked crab meat

2 eggs, lightly beaten

1 tblspn chopped chives

1 Heat the oil in a large frying pan over moderate heat. Add the spring onions, pimentos and bacon, cook for 3 minutes, remove from heat.

2 Heat the soup and stock in a large saucepan, add dissolved cornflour, cook over moderate heat, stirring constantly, until soup begins to thicken.

3 Add the crab meat, spring onions, pimentos and bacon, cook for a further 1 minute.

4 Just before serving, stir in the beaten eggs and garnish with chopped chives.

Serves 4

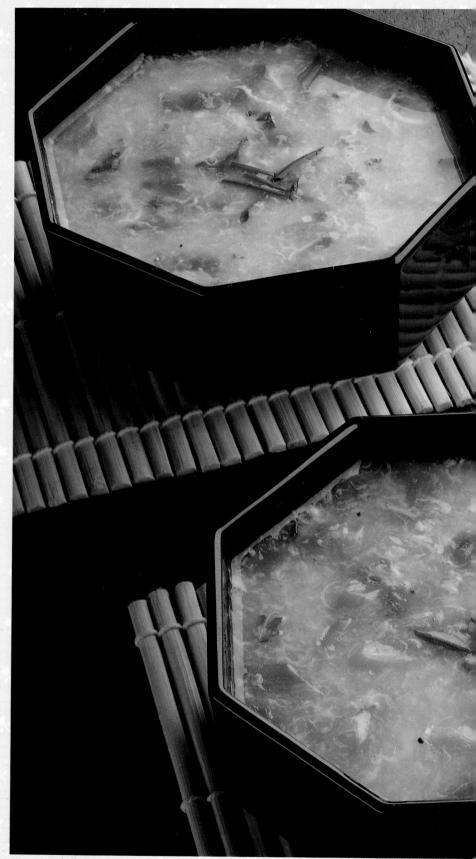

Crab Soup

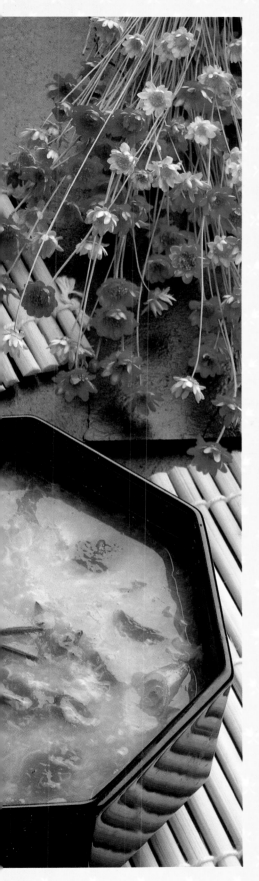

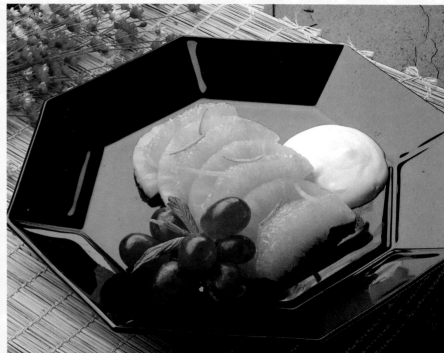

Oriental Oranges with Yoghurt

Oriental Oranges with Yoghurt

544 kilojoules/130 calories per serving

2 tblspn castor sugar

¼ cup freshly squeezed orange juice

1 tblspn freshly squeezed lime juice

2 tspn lime rind, cut into thin strips

2 tspn orange rind, cut into thin strips

8 tinned, unsweetened pineapple rings, halved

2 oranges, peeled and segmented

½ cup plain natural yoghurt

4 small bunches of red grapes

mint sprigs for garnish

1 In a small saucepan, heat the sugar, orange juice and lime juice until simmering. Add the lime and orange rind, cook for 5 minutes, remove syrup from heat.

2 Arrange the pineapple and orange segments on each of 4 serving plates and pour a tablespoon of syrup over each serving of fruit.

3 Serve with yoghurt and small bunch of grapes. Garnish with fresh sprig of mint if desired.

Serves 4

WINTER DINNER

*Fresh Parmesan Cheese Salad
with Croutons*

*Bacon and Bean Casserole
with Barley*

Red Cabbage with Caraway Seeds

Tangy Pear and Raspberry Cobbler

Fresh Parmesan Cheese Salad with Croutons

1068 kilojoules/255 calories per serving

30g (1oz) lite margarine

4 slices white bread, crusts removed

1 curly endive, torn into bite-size pieces

125g (4oz) Parmesan cheese, cut into small pieces

1 red capsicum (pepper), seeded, cut into short thin strips

1 tblspn freshly squeezed lemon juice

1 tblspn olive oil

2 cloves garlic, crushed

2 tblspn freshly squeezed orange juice

1 Melt the margarine in a small frying pan over low heat. Cut the bread into small triangles and add to the frying pan. Cook, turning frequently until golden, drain on a paper towel.

2 Arrange the endive, cheese and capsicum strips on a serving plate.

3 In a small bowl, mix together the lemon juice, olive oil, garlic and orange juice. Pour over salad, sprinkle croutons on top and serve immediately.

Serves 4

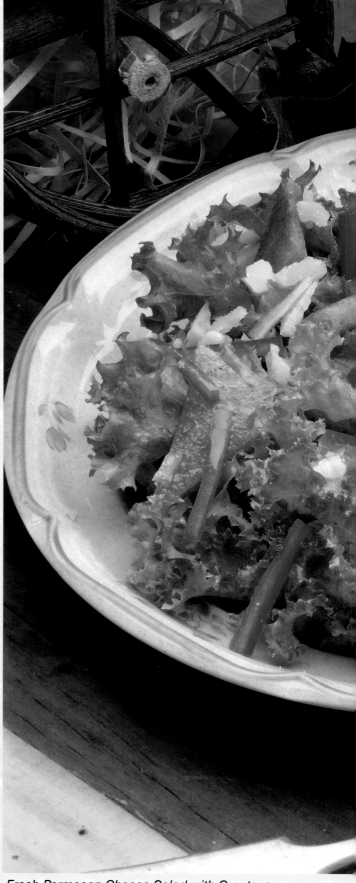

Fresh Parmesan Cheese Salad with Croutons

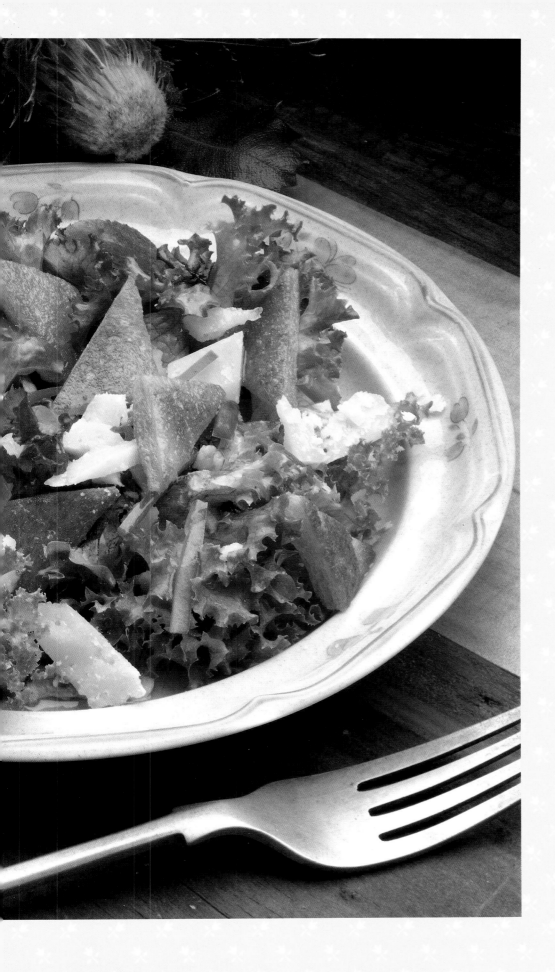

Bacon and Bean Casserole with Barley

1110 kilojoules/265 calories per serving

1 cup barley

1 tblspn oil

2 onions, chopped

6 lean bacon rashers, rind and fat removed, chopped

¼ tspn cinnamon

1 tspn chopped fresh thyme

100g (3½oz) button mushrooms, sliced

1½ cups red kidney beans, rinsed and drained

1½ cups tinned tomatoes

1 cup tomato puree

1 tblspn chopped fresh parsley

1 Bring a large saucepan of water to the boil, add the barley, cook until tender, about 30 minutes.

2 Heat the oil in a large frying pan over moderate heat. Add the onions and bacon, cook for 4 minutes. Add the cinnamon, thyme and mushrooms, cook for a further 3 minutes.

3 Stir in the beans, tomatoes and tomato puree, cover and simmer for 30 minutes, stirring occasionally.

4 Stir in the parsley and serve with the barley.

Serves 4

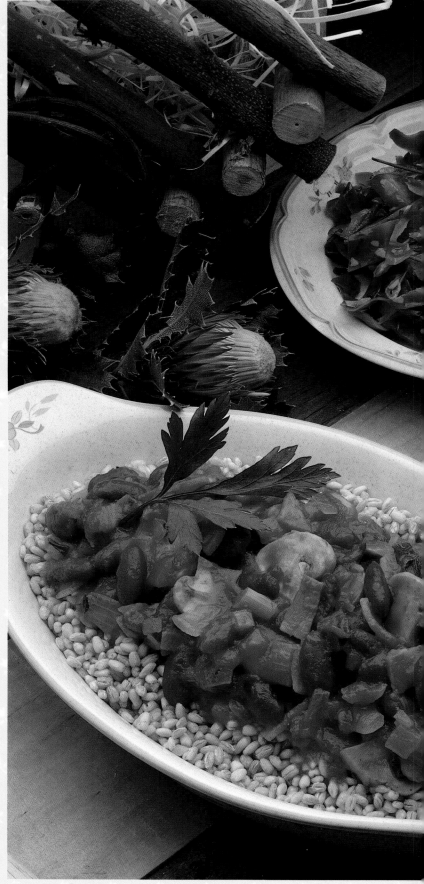

Top: Red Cabbage with Caraway Seeds.
Bottom: Bacon and Bean Casserole with Barley

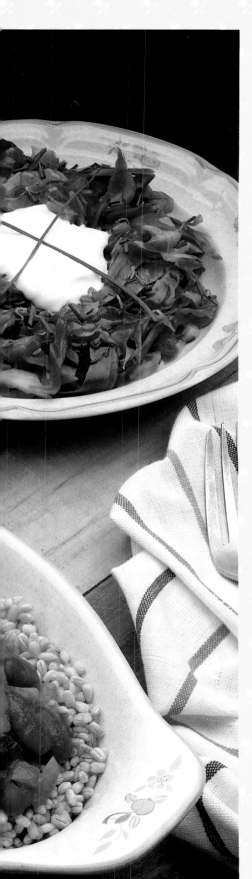

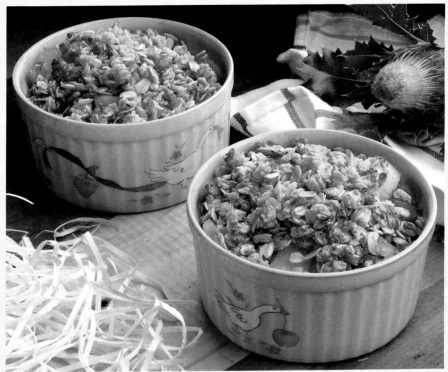

Red Cabbage with Caraway Seeds

188 kilojoules/45 calories per serving

½ medium red cabbage

2 tblspn red wine vinegar

2 tspn caraway seeds

¼ tspn nutmeg

¼ cup roughly chopped chives

1 tblspn lite sour cream

1 tblspn natural low fat yoghurt

chives to garnish

1 Wash the cabbage and place in a saucepan with 3cm (1¼ in) of boiling water. Add the vinegar, caraway seeds and nutmeg. Cover and boil for 2-3 minutes. Drain well, toss in the chives.

2 Combine sour cream and yoghurt in a small bowl, serve on top of cabbage, garnish with chives.

Serves 4

Tangy Pear and Raspberry Cobbler

1235 kilojoules/295 calories per serving

4 pears, peeled, cored

1 tblspn lemon juice

1 cup fresh raspberries

1 tblspn lite margarine

1 tblspn brown sugar

¾ cup unsweetened toasted muesli

1 Sprinkle the pears with lemon juice and cut into 1cm (½in) pieces. Arrange raspberries and pieces of pear in four ½-cup capacity ramekins.

2 Melt the margarine in a medium saucepan, add the sugar and muesli, mix well.

3 Spoon mixture on top of each ramekin, bake in moderate oven for 15 minutes.

Serves 4

MEDITERRANEAN DINNER

Pimento and Tomato Soup

Eggplant (Aubergine) and Mint Bake

*Poached Tuna with Rosemary on
Blanched Asparagus*

*Fresh Berry Compote in Yoghurt
Brandy Sauce*

Eggplant (Aubergine) and Mint Bake

628 kilojoules/150 calories per serving

2 eggplants (aubergine), cut into 1cm (½in) cubes

3 tomatoes, chopped

2 cloves garlic, crushed

2 tblspn chopped fresh mint

1 tblspn olive oil

60g (2oz) mozzarella cheese, grated

4 tblspn grated Parmesan cheese

1 Toss the eggplant with 2 tablespoons salt. Set aside for 30 minutes. Rinse under cold water and drain.

2 In a medium bowl, combine the eggplant, tomatoes, garlic, mint and olive oil, toss well. Spoon mixture into an ovenproof baking dish, sprinkle with the combined mozzarella and Parmesan cheeses.

3 Bake in a moderate oven for 45 minutes, or until eggplant is very tender.

Serves 4

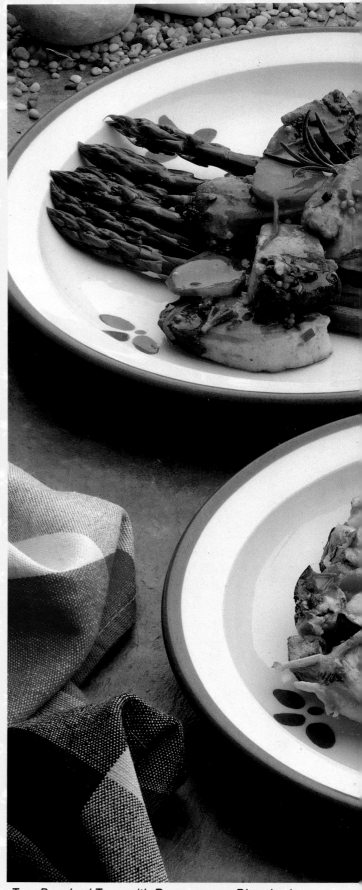

Top: Poached Tuna with Rosemary on Blanched Asparagus. Bottom: Eggplant (Aubergine) and Mint Bake

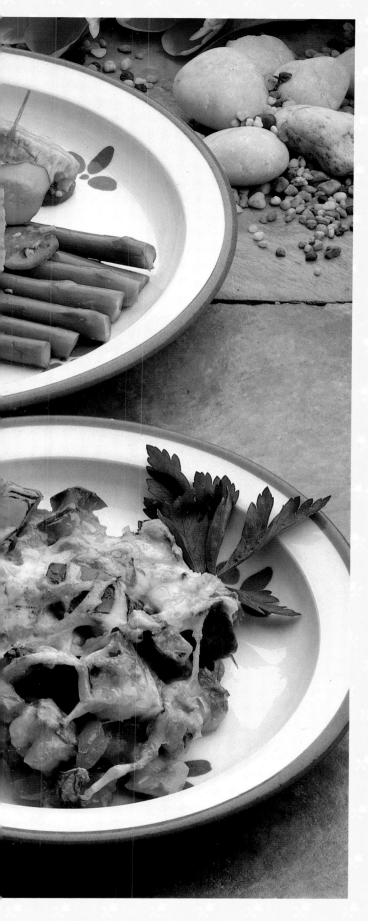

Poached Tuna with Rosemary on Blanched Asparagus

795 kilojoules/190 calories per serving

1 cup dry white wine

3 tblspn red wine vinegar

¼ cup freshly squeezed lime juice

1 tspn yellow mustard seeds

½ tspn cracked black pepper

1 tspn sambal oelek (chilli paste)

1 tblspn chopped fresh rosemary

2 tblspn red capsicum (pepper), cut into thin strips

625g (1lb 4oz) tuna fillet, cut into 2cm (¾in) cubes

1 large bunch asparagus, trimmed

1 Heat the wine, red wine vinegar, ½ cup water and lime juice in a medium frying pan over moderate heat until simmering.

2 Add the mustard seeds, black pepper, sambal oelek, rosemary, capsicum strips and tuna pieces. Cook tuna until cooked through, about 5 minutes.

3 Meanwhile, bring a large saucepan of water to the boil, add the asparagus and cook for 1½ to 2 minutes or until just cooked. Refresh under cold running water, drain.

4 Divide the asparagus between plates. Remove the tuna with a slotted spoon and arrange over top of the asparagus.

5 Reheat the tuna poaching liquid until simmering, cook until sauce is reduced by half. Pour over tuna, serve immediately.

Serves 4

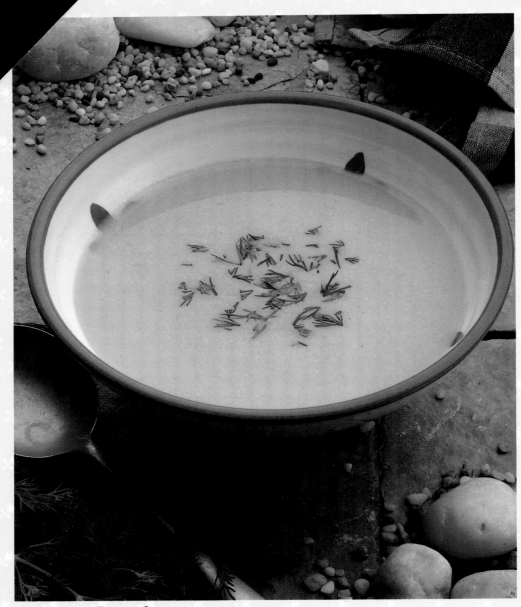

Pimento and Tomato Soup

Pimento and Tomato Soup

461 kilojoules/110 calories per serving

2 tspn olive oil

¾ cup chopped lean ham

1 onion, finely chopped

3 cups pimento, drained and chopped

2 cups degreased chicken or vegetable stock

2 tblspn tomato paste

2 tspn castor sugar

½ tspn ground nutmeg

4 tblspn lite cream cheese

1 tblspn arrowroot dissolved in 2 tblspn water

1 tblspn chopped fresh dill

1 Heat the oil in a medium frying pan, add the ham, onion and pimentos, cook for 5 minutes.

2 Add the stock, tomato paste, sugar and nutmeg, cook for a further 5 minutes. Puree the mixture and cream cheese in a blender or food processor for 3 minutes, pour mixture through a sieve.

3 Pour mixture into a large saucepan, add dissolved arrowroot and cook over moderate heat, stirring constantly until slightly thickened.

4 Serve hot and sprinkle chopped dill on top for garnish.

Serves 4

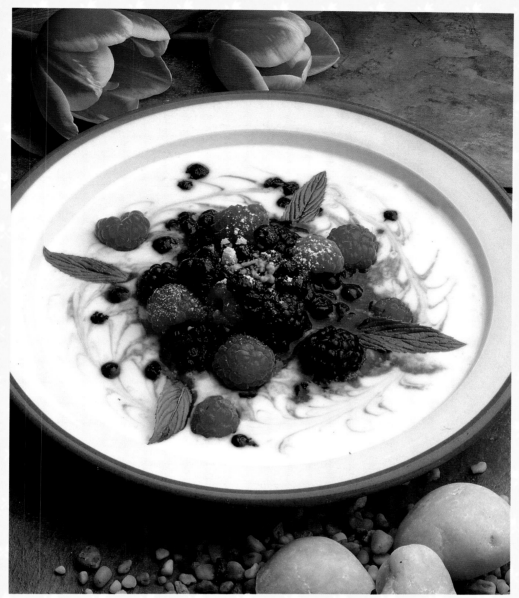

Fresh Berry Compote in Yoghurt Brandy Sauce

Fresh Berry Compote in Yoghurt Brandy Sauce

628 kilojoules/150 calories per serving

½ cup natural low fat yoghurt

2 tblspn lite cream cheese, softened

1 tspn vanilla essence

1 tblspn brandy

1 cup tinned wild blueberries, reserve liquid

¾ cup fresh raspberries

½ cup mulberries

1 tblspn icing sugar, for dusting

16 mint leaves for decoration

1 In a small bowl, combine the yogurt, cream cheese, vanilla essence and brandy, mix well. Divide the mixture onto each flat serving plate and smooth out with a spoon.

2 Spoon 1 tablespoon of the reserved blueberry juice onto the centre of the cream. Using a skewer, draw the blueberry liquid through the cream, to make a pattern.

3 Spoon a small pile of the combined raspberries, blueberries and mulberries in the centre of each plate. Sprinkle with icing sugar and decorate with fresh mint leaves.

Serves 4

VEGETARIAN LUNCH

Fennel and Orange Salad with Orange Vinaigrette

Cheesy Rice Ring with Garlic Vegetables

Spicy Bean and Vegetable Salad

Lemon and Basil Granita

Fennel and Orange Salad with Orange Vinaigrette

272 kilojoules/65 calories per serving

8 butter lettuce leaves

¾ cup sliced fennel, white part only

½ red capsicum (pepper), finely sliced into short strips

2 tblspn finely sliced orange rind

½ cup fresh basil leaves, cut into thin strips

2 oranges, segmented

2 tblspn freshly squeezed orange juice

2 tblspn white wine vinegar

2 tblspn low-joule French dressing

1 Arrange two lettuce leaves on each salad plate.

2 In a medium bowl, combine the fennel, capsicum, orange rind, basil and orange segments.

3 Pour over the combined orange juice, vinegar and French dressing, toss well.

4 Divide the salad in four and place on the lettuce leaves.

Serves 4

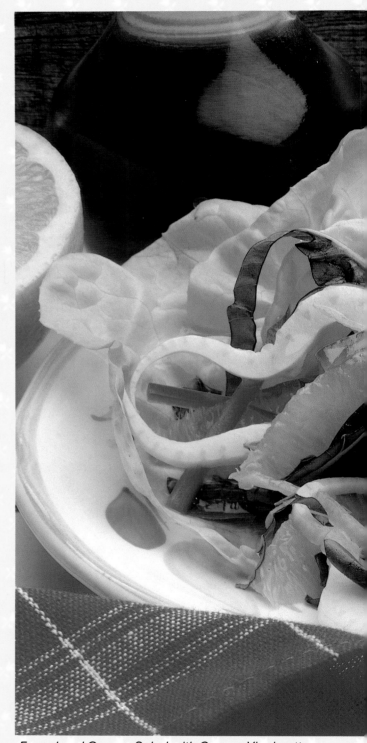

Fennel and Orange Salad with Orange Vinaigrette

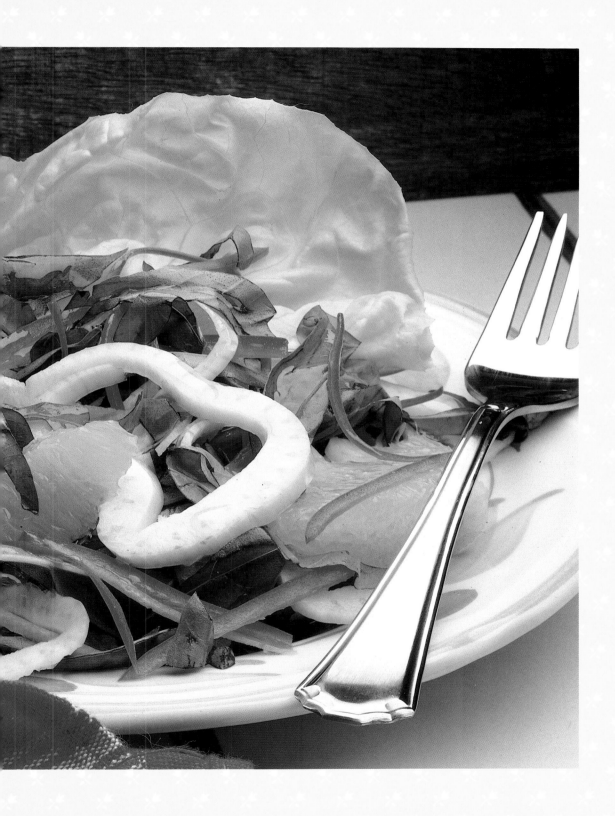

Cheesy Rice Ring with Garlic Vegetables

837 kilojoules/200 calories per serving

2½ cups cooked long grain white rice

60g (2oz) fresh Parmesan cheese, finely grated

1 tblspn olive oil

2 tspn olive oil, extra

3 cloves garlic, crushed

1 red capsicum (pepper), seeded and cut into 1cm (½in) squares

1 green capsicum (pepper), seeded and cut into 1cm (½in) squares

1 cup oyster mushrooms

1 tblspn chopped Italian parsley

1 Place the cooked rice into a large bowl. Stir in the cheese and olive oil, mix well. Spoon the rice into a lightly oiled ring mould and press down firmly.

2 Cover the mould with foil and bake in a moderate oven for 10 minutes.

3 Heat the extra olive oil in a large frying pan. Add the garlic and cook for 3 minutes. Add the capsicum, mushrooms and parsley, cook, stirring constantly for 4 minutes.

4 Turn the rice ring out onto a serving plate, fill with the garlic vegetables.

Serves 4

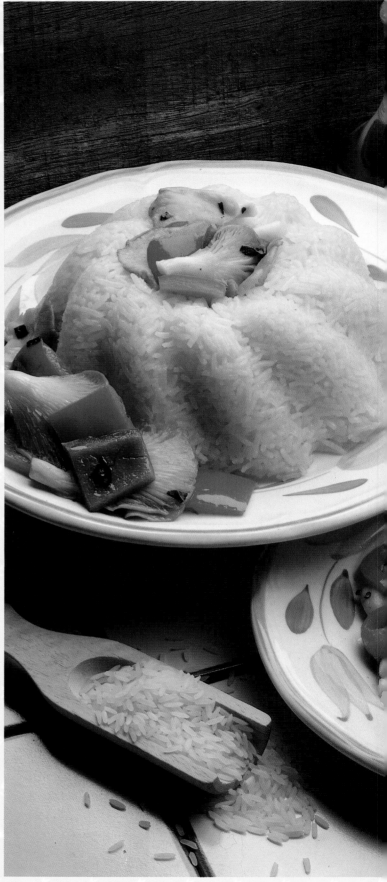

Top: Cheesy Rice Ring with Garlic Vegetables.
Bottom: Spicy Bean and Vegetable Salad

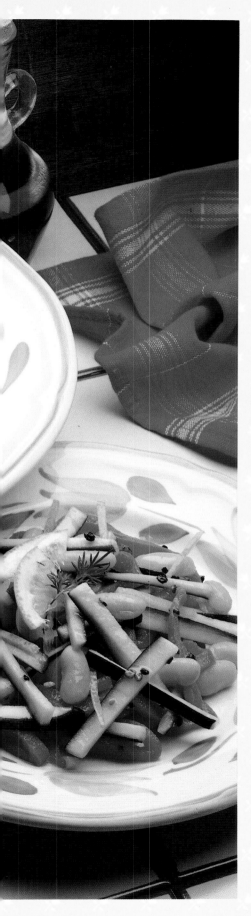

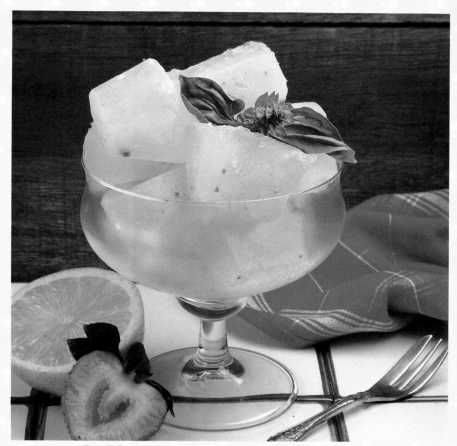

Lemon and Basil Granita

Spicy Bean and Vegetable Salad

377 kilojoules/90 calories per serving

1 cup butter beans, rinsed and drained

2 zucchini (courgette), cut into thin strips

1 cup pimentos, drained, cut into strips

¼ tspn cracked black pepper

½ tspn sambal oelek (chilli paste)

1 tblspn olive oil

1 tblspn freshly squeezed lemon juice

1 Arrange the butter beans, zucchini strips and pimento strips on a serving plate.

2 In a small bowl, combine the cracked black pepper, sambal oelek, olive oil and lemon juice, mix well.

3 Pour over salad and garnish with fresh lemon slices and a sprig of dill if desired.

Serves 4

Lemon and Basil Granita

335 kilojoules/80 calories per serving

2 cups sweet white wine

1 cup basil leaves, chopped

¼ cup castor sugar

1 cup freshly squeezed lemon juice

1 tblspn grated lemon rind

3 tblspn freshly squeezed lime juice

1 Combine the wine, basil and sugar in a small saucepan over moderate heat. Bring to the boil, cook for 3 minutes.

2 Pour mixture through a sieve to strain, cool liquid. When liquid is at room temperature, stir in the lemon juice, lemon rind and lime juice.

3 Pour mixture into an ice tray and freeze. Remove a few minutes before serving and spoon into dessert glasses. Decorate with fresh basil and strawberries if desired.

Serves 4

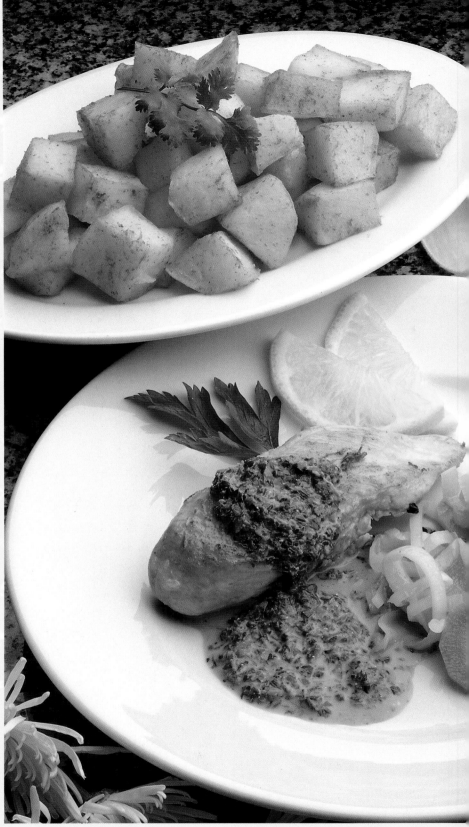

CELEBRATION DINNER

Mussels in Wine and Tomato Sauce

Chicken Breasts with Green Sauce

Spicy Baked Potatoes

Fluffy Blueberry Mousse

Chicken Breasts with Green Sauce

837 kilojoules/200 calories per serving

1 tblspn lite margarine

4 single chicken breast fillets

1 cup Italian parsley leaves

¾ cup basil leaves

1 clove garlic, crushed

2 tspn capers, drained

1 tblspn olive oil

2 tblspn red wine vinegar

2 tblspn degreased chicken stock

1 tblspn freshly squeezed lime juice

1 tblspn low fat plain yoghurt

1 Heat the margarine in a medium frying pan over moderate heat. Add the chicken fillets, cook, turning frequently until golden and cooked through, about 3 minutes each side.

2 In a food processor or blender, process the parsley, basil, garlic, capers, olive oil, red wine vinegar, chicken stock and lime juice for 2 minutes.

3 Pour into a small saucepan and heat quickly, stir in the yoghurt and serve over chicken breasts. Serve with fresh blanched carrots and leeks.

Serves 4

Top: Spicy Baked Potatoes. Bottom: Chicken Breasts with Green Sauce

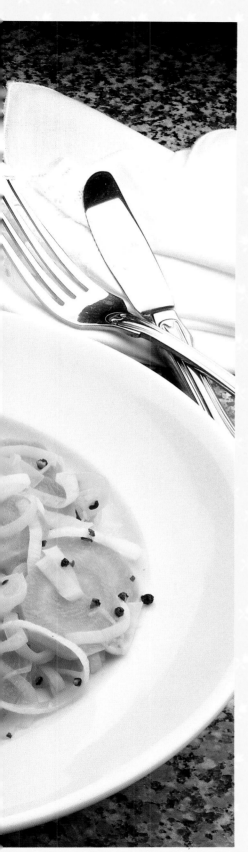

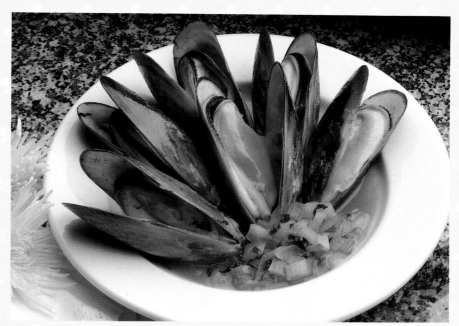

Mussels in Wine and Tomato Sauce

Spicy Baked Potatoes

502 kilojoules/120 calories per serving

4 medium potatoes, peeled, cut into 1cm (½in) cubes

1 tspn ground cumin

1 tspn ground coriander

½ tspn salt

¼ tspn ground chilli powder

¼ tspn ground paprika

2 tspn oil

1 Bring a large saucepan of water to the boil, add the potato cubes and parboil for 5 minutes.

2 Drain potatoes and toss in the combined cumin, coriander, salt, chilli and paprika.

3 Brush a baking dish with the oil, add the potatoes and bake in a moderate oven for 20-25 minutes, or until cooked through, stirring occasionally.

Serves 4

Mussels in Wine and Tomato Sauce

502 kilojoules/120 calories per serving

1 tblspn lite margarine

1 large onion, chopped

4 cloves garlic, crushed

1 tblspn finely chopped red capsicum (pepper)

1 cup dry white wine

2 tblspn low-joule French Dressing

1 tblspn tomato paste

24 mussels, scrubbed and debearded

1 tblspn finely chopped fresh basil

1 Melt the margarine in a large frying pan over moderate heat. Add the onion and garlic, cook for 2 minutes.

2 Add the capsicum, wine, French dressing and tomato paste, cook for a further 1 minute.

3 Add the mussels, cover and simmer for 3-5 minutes or until the mussels open. Remove mussels with a slotted spoon, discard any that do not open.

4 Cook the sauce for a further 3 minutes, or until it thickens slightly. Stir in the basil and pour the sauce over the mussels, serve immediately.

Serves 4

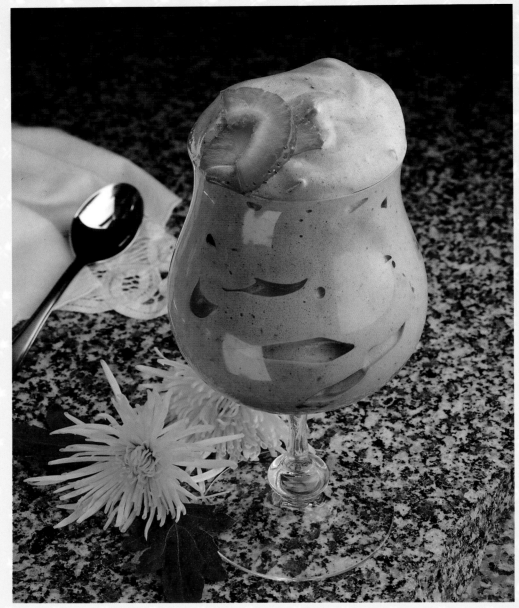

Fluffy Blueberry Mousse

Fluffy Blueberry Mousse

628 kilojoules/150 calories per serving

1½ cups blueberries (can use tinned blueberries)

2 tblspn freshly squeezed lemon juice

1 tblspn arrowroot, dissolved in 2 tblspn water

3 egg-whites

¼ cup castor sugar

strawberry slices for garnish

1 Place the blueberries and lemon juice in a medium saucepan over moderate heat. Add 2 tablespoons water and bring to the boil. Stir in the dissolved arrowroot, remove from heat, push mixture through a sieve or puree. Cool to room temperature.

2 Beat the egg-whites with the sugar until soft peaks form. Beat the cooled blueberry puree into the egg-whites and spoon into serving glasses.

3 Serve immediately as mixture will separate if left to stand for over 1 hour. Decorate with fresh strawberries if desired.

Serves 4

OVER 60 SNACKS UNDER 50 CALORIES (210 KILOJOULES)

- 3 king prawns (shrimp)
- 8 raw oysters
- ½ hard-boiled egg
- 1 chocolate chip biscuit
- 20 thin pretzel sticks
- ½ celery stalk stuffed with 2 teaspoons peanut butter
- 1 celery stalk stuffed with 1 tablespoon camembert
- 3 small dried apricot halves spread with 2 teaspoons melted dark chocolate
- ¼ cup dry white wine mixed with ¼ cup soda water
- ⅓ cup grape juice mixed with ⅓ cup soda water, served over ice, garnished with a strip of lemon
- ⅓ cup apricot nectar
- ⅓ cup cider
- ¾ cup popped corn, tossed with ¾ teaspoon melted butter or margarine, ¾ teaspoon freshly grated Parmesan cheese, and a pinch of cayenne powder
- 2 tablespoons low fat cottage cheese, sprinkled with 2 teaspoons raisins
- ½ cup chopped apple sprinkled with ½ teaspoon dessicated coconut
- ½ cup canned water-packed fruit cocktail
- ¾ cup fresh strawberries topped with 2 teaspoons low fat yoghurt
- ½ a medium orange sprinkled with 2 teaspoons dessicated coconut
- ½ cup fresh blueberries
- 4 fresh passionfruit
- ½ a pear
- 2 yellow plums
- 1 cup chopped watermelon
- ⅓ cup seedless grapes

- ½ cup chopped fresh pineapple
- ¾ cup honeydew melon cubes topped with 3 teaspoons vanilla yoghurt
- ½ a medium grapefruit drizzled with 1 teaspoon honey
- 6 slices cucumber spread with 2 tablespoons French onion dip
- 3 medium fresh apricots
- 1 small apple
- 1 small ladyfinger banana
- ½ a small rockmelon (cantaloupe)
- 5 fresh lychees
- 10 cherries
- 1 fresh peach
- 1 small orange
- 2 small nectarines
- 2 small mandarines
- 1 kiwi fruit
- 4 dates
- 2 small dried figs
- 3 prunes
- 5 small dried peach halves
- 8 beer nuts
- 5 cashews
- 10 dry roasted cashews
- 3 pecans
- 7 pistachios
- 4 half walnuts
- 7 shelled almonds
- 3 sugared almonds
- 2 macadamia nuts
- 2 brazil nuts
- 10 hazelnuts
- 15 black olives
- 16 green olives
- 5 pickled onions
- 2 artichokes with freshly squeezed lemon juice
- 2 large raw carrots
- 16 fresh asparagus spears
- 16 cherry tomatoes
- 1 cup cauliflowerets drizzled with 2 teaspoons low-joule salad dressing

Fibre in Your Slimming Plan

Fibre plays an important role in helping reduce your weight. The added advantage of eating a high fibre diet is almost certainly a lowering of blood cholesterol levels.

Foods high in fibre

Grains	brown rice bulgur wholemeal pasta wheatgerm unprocessed bran oatbran
Cereals	oatbran All-Bran Shredded Wheat Old-fashioned oatmeal
Fruit	orange grapefruit } don't removed mandarine } membranes apples pears peaches } don't remove skin grapes
Dried Fruit	apricots prunes apples raisins
Vegetables	dried beans and peas celery carrots broccoli green beans peas cabbage asparagus cauliflower corn
Raw vegetables	celery carrot broccoli cucumber zucchini lettuce

MEAT

Meat is an important part of our diet, even when we are watching our weight. It is an excellent source of protein, vitamins and minerals.

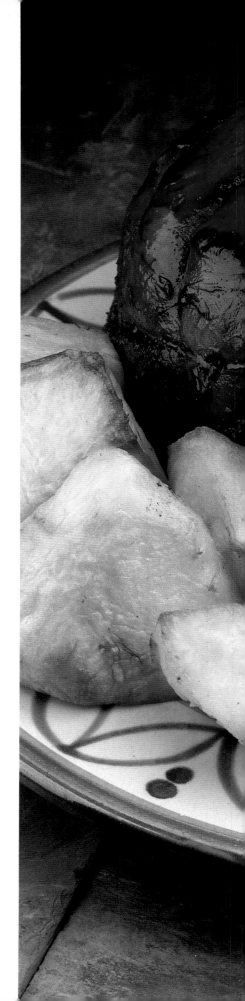

Green Peppercorn Steak with Mustard Sauce

1151 kilojoules/275 calories per serving

3 tblspn green peppercorns, drained

6 rib-eye beef steaks, 155g (5oz) each

SAUCE

1 carton thick yoghurt

1 tblspn hot English mustard

2 tblspn chopped parsley

salt

1 Crush peppercorns with the blade of a knife, press into both sides of the steaks.

2 To make the sauce: Combine yoghurt, mustard and parsley in a bowl, stir until well combined. Season to taste with salt. Cover, refrigerate.

3 Heat griller, place steaks on a lightly oiled griller tray. Cook 6 minutes, turning once, for medium rare.

4 Serve on heated plates with the mustard sauce.

Serves 6

Roasted Veal with Honey Glaze

1507 kilojoules/360 calories per serving

1.5kg (3lb) nut of veal

2 tblspn apricot jam

1 tblspn honey

2 tblspn soy sauce

¼ cup freshly squeezed lemon juice

2 tblspn red wine vinegar

1 tspn cracked black pepper

1 Secure veal with string and place in a shallow baking dish.

2 Combine the jam, honey, soy sauce, lemon juice, red wine vinegar and black pepper in a small saucepan over low heat, stir until well combined.

3 Brush the veal with the glaze and bake in a moderate oven for 1½ hours. Baste the veal with the glaze every 15 minutes.

4 Slice meat and serve with roasted vegetables.

Serves 8

Roasted Veal with Honey Glaze

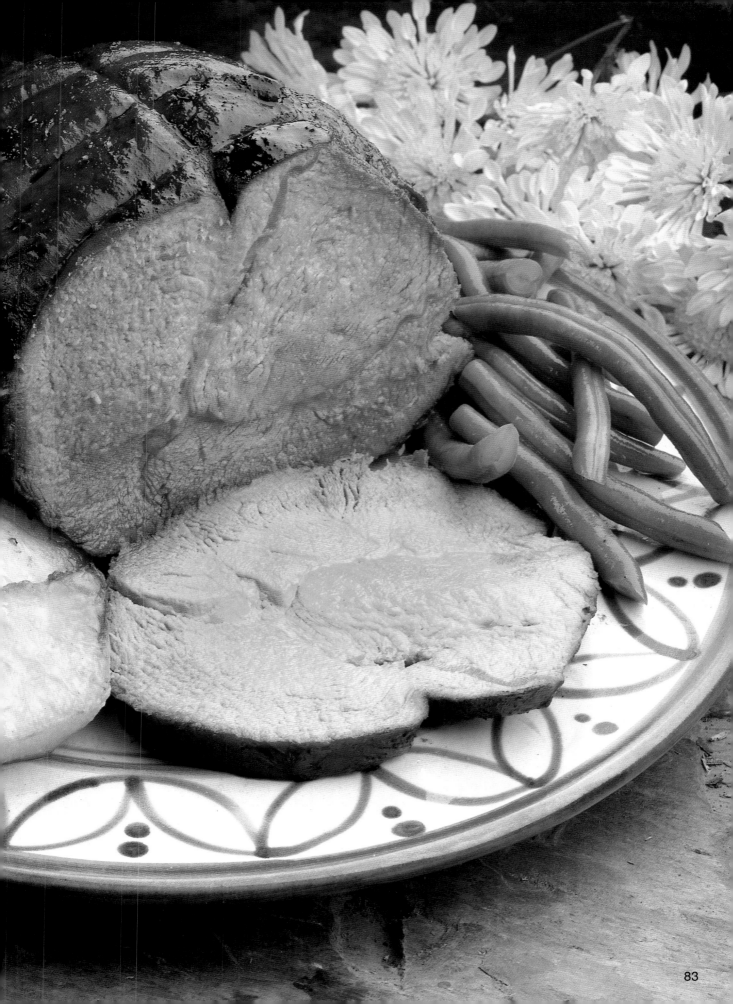

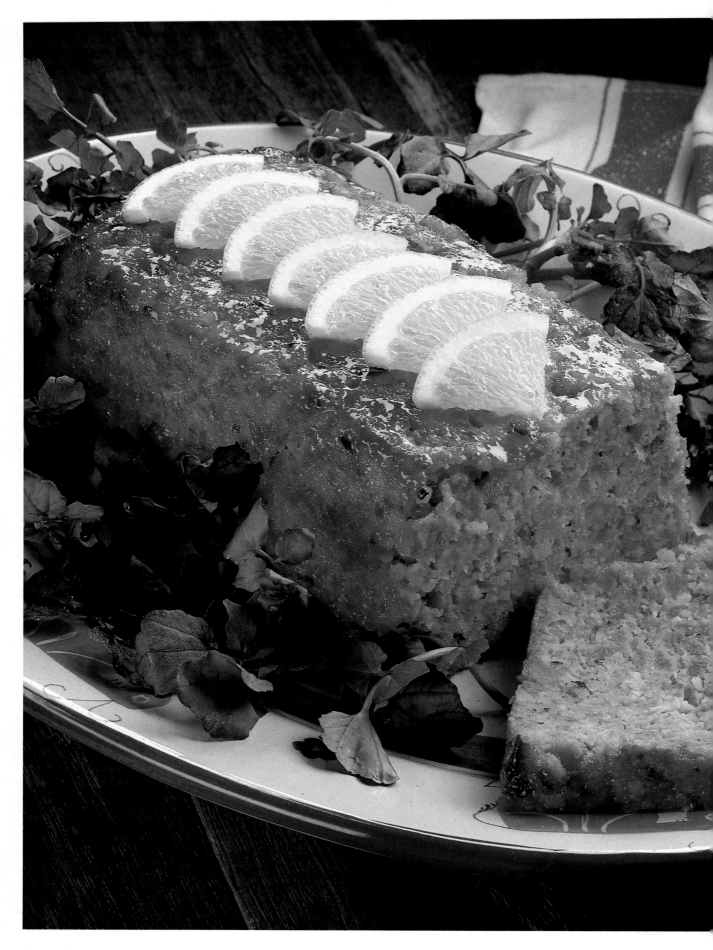

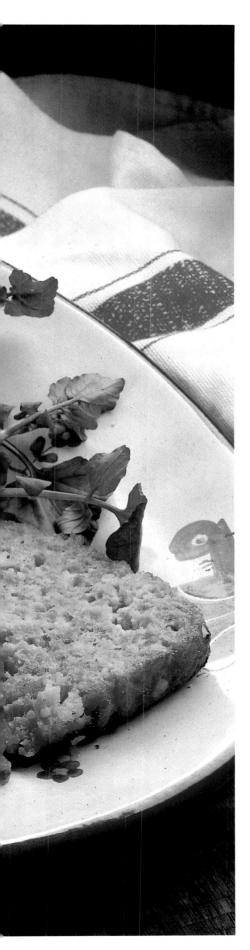

Lamb Rissoles with Cucumber Sauce

816 kilojoules/195 calories per serving (2 rissoles each)

625g (1lb 4oz) lean lamb, any visible fat removed, roughly chopped

2 slices bread, crusts removed, quartered

1 onion, roughly chopped

1 clove garlic, chopped

2 egg-whites

1 tblspn chopped fresh mint

2 tspn white wine vinegar

salt

pepper

1 tblspn olive oil

CUCUMBER SAUCE

1 cucumber, peeled, seeded, finely chopped

150ml (¼ pint) degreased chicken stock

⅓ cup plain yogurt

2 tspn cornflour

2 tblspn chopped fresh mint

salt

1 Combine lamb, bread, onion, garlic, egg-whites, mint and vinegar in a processor. Process until finely minced. Season to taste with salt and freshly ground pepper.

2 Divide mixture into 12 balls, flatten into patties, place on a platter, cover and refrigerate for at least 1 hour.

3 Heat oil in a large non-stick frying pan, cook rissoles in batches until brown all over, about 12 minutes, turning once. Keep rissoles warm on a heated platter.

4 Add cucumber to the frying pan, saute 1 minute. Add stock, bring to a boil, reduce heat, simmer 3 minutes.

5 In a small bowl whisk yoghurt and cornflour together, add ¼ cup of the hot stock, then tip contents of the bowl into the frying pan, stir over gentle heat until heated through.

6 Add mint, season to taste with salt and freshly ground white pepper. Serve sauce separately with the hot rissoles.

Serves 6

Glazed Ham and Pork Loaf

1172 kilojoules/280 calories per serving

375g (¾lb) lean ham

½ cup dried apricots

500g (1lb) pork mince

3 tblspn chopped parsley

1 cup dry breadcrumbs

1¼ cup skim milk

½ cup brown sugar

3 tblspn apple cider vinegar

2 tblspn Dijon mustard

1 In a food processor or blender, process the ham and apricots until finely chopped.

2 Place pork in a large mixing bowl, add the ham and apricot mixture, parsley, breadcrumbs and skim milk, mix well.

3 Press mixture into a greased and lined loaf tin. Bake in a moderate oven for 15 minutes.

4 Meanwhile, mix together the sugar, vinegar, mustard and ¼ cup water in a small saucepan over moderate heat. Bring to the boil, reduce heat and simmer for 10-15 minutes. Remove from heat.

5 Brush top of loaf with some of the glaze, return to oven for another 15 minutes, glaze again, repeat every 15 minutes until loaf has been in oven for 1 hour.

6 Turn loaf out onto a baking tray, brush glaze over bottom and sides, cook for a further 15 minutes. Cool for 15 minutes before slicing.

Makes 10 slices

Glazed Ham and Pork Loaf

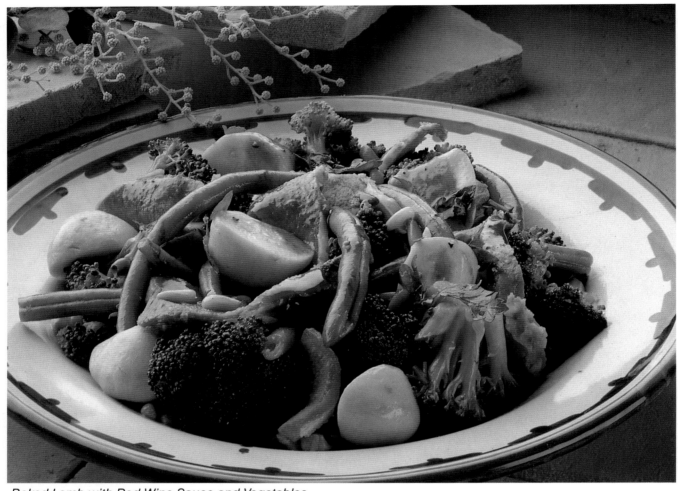

Baked Lamb with Red Wine Sauce and Vegetables

Baked Lamb with Red Wine Sauce and Vegetables

1340 kilojoules/320 calories per serving

1kg (2lb) boned and rolled loin of lamb

2 tblspn redcurrant jelly

½ cup red wine

2 tspn finely chopped fresh rosemary

¾ cup yellow squash, sliced

250g (½lb) green beans, tops and tails removed

1 cup broccoli flowerets

2 tblspn chopped Italian parsley

1 Place the lamb in an ovenproof dish, bake in moderate oven for 15 minutes.

2 In a small saucepan, combine the redcurrant jelly with the red wine and rosemary over moderate heat and bring to the boil.

3 Pour half the red wine sauce mixture over the meat and return to the oven for a further 45 minutes, basting regularly with the pan juices.

4 Meanwhile, bring a large saucepan of water to the boil, add the squash, beans and broccoli and cook for 1 minute. Remove vegetables with a slotted spoon and refresh under cold water. Arrange on a serving plate.

5 Remove lamb from oven when cooked, slice and arrange with the vegetables.

6 Pour the pan juices into the saucepan with the remaining red wine sauce mixture. Bring to the boil, reduce heat and simmer until sauce thickens slightly. Sprinkle the parsley over lamb and pour sauce over the top.

Serves 4

Osso Buco with Vegetables

1800 kilojoules/430 calories per serving

1 tblspn olive oil

1kg (2lb) veal shanks, sliced

¾ cup dry white wine

1 onion, sliced

3 zucchini (courgette), sliced

2 carrots, sliced

2 stalks celery, sliced

2 cloves garlic, crushed

1½ cups chicken stock

425g (13½oz) can tomato puree

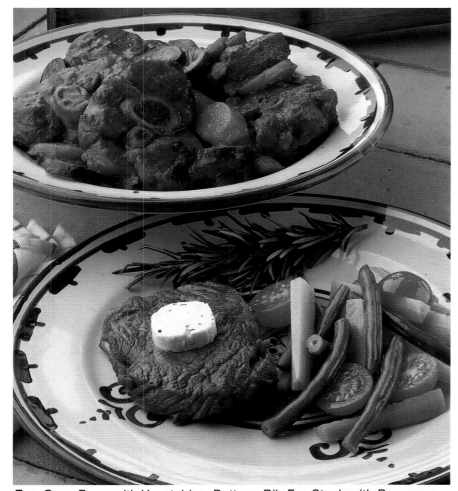

Top: Osso Buco with Vegetables. Bottom: Rib Eye Steak with Rosemary Cheese Butter

1 Heat the oil in a very large, deep (preferably non-stick) frying pan, over moderate heat. Add the veal and brown on all sides. Stir in the wine and bring to the boil.

2 Add the onion, zucchini, carrot, celery, garlic, stock and tomato puree. Reduce heat and cook until liquid is reduced by half, stirring occasionally.

3 Add ½ cup water and continue to cook for 1 hour or until meat is tender. You may have to add extra water if sauce gets too thick.

Serves 4

Rib Eye Steak with Rosemary Cheese Butter

1089 kilojoules/260 calories per serving
45g (1½oz) lite margarine
1 tblspn butter
45g (1½oz) cream cheese
2 tspn rosemary, finely chopped
1 clove garlic, crushed
4 rib eye steaks, 155g (5oz) each

1 Soften margarine, butter and cream cheese to room temperature. Mix until well combined, mix in rosemary and garlic. Spoon mixture onto a piece of foil and roll up into a sausage shape, freeze until ready to serve.

2 Grill steaks on a rack until just cooked. Slice frozen cheese and butter roll into ½cm (¼in) slices and place one slice on top of each steak.

Serves 4

Thai Pork Fillet Salad

1047 kilojoules/250 calories per serving
⅓ cup degreased chicken stock
1½ tblspn tamari (see note)
⅓ cup freshly squeezed lemon juice
2 cloves garlic, finely chopped
1 tspn dark brown sugar
pepper
½ tspn chilli flakes
⅓ cup chopped fresh coriander
845g (1lb 11oz) pork fillet, any visible fat removed
500g (1lb) cucumber, very thinly sliced
1 onion, thinly sliced, separated into rings
440g (14oz) radish, very thinly sliced
2 tblspn safflower oil

1 In a bowl, combine stock, tamari, 2 tablespoons of the lemon juice, garlic, sugar, freshly ground pepper to taste, chilli flakes and 2 tablespoons of the coriander. Pour over pork fillet, cover, marinate overnight in refrigerator, or for 2 hours at room temperature. Baste and turn from time to time.

2 Combine cucumber, onion and radish in a bowl. Set aside.

3 When ready to cook, remove pork from marinade, dry with paper towels. Set aside.

4 Strain marinade into a small saucepan, bring to a boil. Remove from the heat, stir in oil and remaining 2 tablespoons lemon juice; pour over vegetables in bowl, add remaining coriander, toss well.

5 Place pork fillets under a pre-heated grill on a lightly oiled griller tray. Cook until medium rare, about 12 minutes, turning once. Allow to rest at room temperature for 5 minutes before carving into thin slices.

6 Remove vegetables from bowl with a slotted spoon, place on a platter. Arrange pork slices on top, pour over any remaining marinade. Serve immediately.

Note: Tamari is like soy sauce, but stronger flavoured. It is available from health food stores.

Serves 6

Dilled Lamb Chops

1298 kilojoules/310 calories per serving

2 tblspn freshly squeezed lemon juice

2 cloves garlic, finely chopped

2 tspn safflower oil

2 tblspn finely chopped fresh dill

8 lamb loin chops, 60g (2oz) each, all visible fat removed

1 Combine lemon juice, garlic, oil and dill in a dish just large enough to hold lamb chops in one layer. Place chops in the dish, turn chops several times to coat with marinade, cover, allow to stand at room temperature for 30-60 minutes.

2 Cook lamb chops under a pre-heated grill until done to your liking, basting with marinade from time to time. Serve hot.

Serves 4

Pork Curry with Cauliflower

1528 kilojoules/365 calories per serving

1 tblspn plain flour

1 tblspn ground coriander

2 tspn ground cumin

¼ tspn chilli flakes

500g (1lb) lean pork leg, cut into 2cm (¾in) cubes

1 tblspn peanut oil

1 onion, chopped

1 red capsicum (pepper), seeded, cut into thin strips

3 cloves garlic, finely chopped

2.5cm (1in) fresh ginger, grated

2 cups degreased stock

juice of 1 lemon

½ cup unsweetened coconut milk

¼ tspn allspice

salt

julienned rind of 1 lemon

185g (6oz) cauliflowerets

1 Combine flour, coriander, cumin and chilli flakes in a small bowl, sprinkle over pork cubes, toss until well coated.

2 Heat oil in a casserole, add pork in batches, saute over medium high heat until brown on all sides. Add onion, capsicum, garlic and ginger, reduce heat, cover, cook for 10 minutes, stirring from time to time.

3 Add stock, lemon juice, coconut milk, allspice and season with salt to taste. Bring to a boil, reduce heat to the barest simmer, cover, cook 45 minutes, or until pork is very nearly tender.

4 Add lemon rind and cauliflowerets, stir in well. Continue simmering until cauliflower is tender, about 12 minutes.

Serves 4

Roast Beef Eye Fillet with Soy Sauce

1507 kilojoules/360 calories per serving

2 tblspn oil

1 tblspn butter

3 tblspn soy sauce

2 tblspn honey

3 tblspn red wine vinegar

1.5kg (3lb) beef eye fillet

3 tspn sesame seeds

1 Heat the oil and butter in a large frying pan. Add the soy sauce, honey and red wine vinegar. Add the fillet and cook over a high heat to sear until brown on all sides.

2 Transfer fillet to an ovenproof dish and bake in a moderate oven for 30-40 minutes or until just cooked. Reserve meat juices and marinade in frying pan.

3 Add the meat juices from the oven dish to the frying pan. Add ¼ cup water and heat over moderate heat until mixture boils.

4 Reduce heat and simmer until mixture thickens, stir in sesame seeds and pour sauce over the sliced meat. Serve with fresh vegetables.

Serves 8

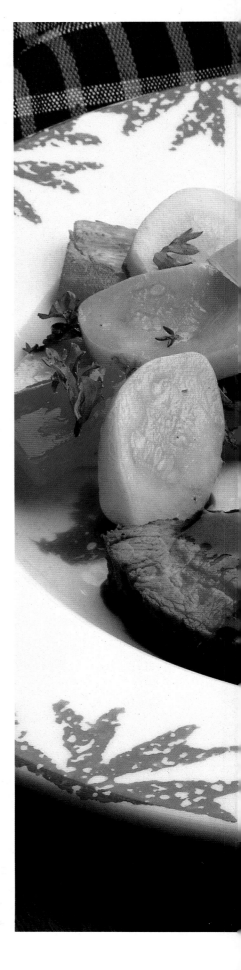

Roast Beef Eye Fillet with Soy Sauce

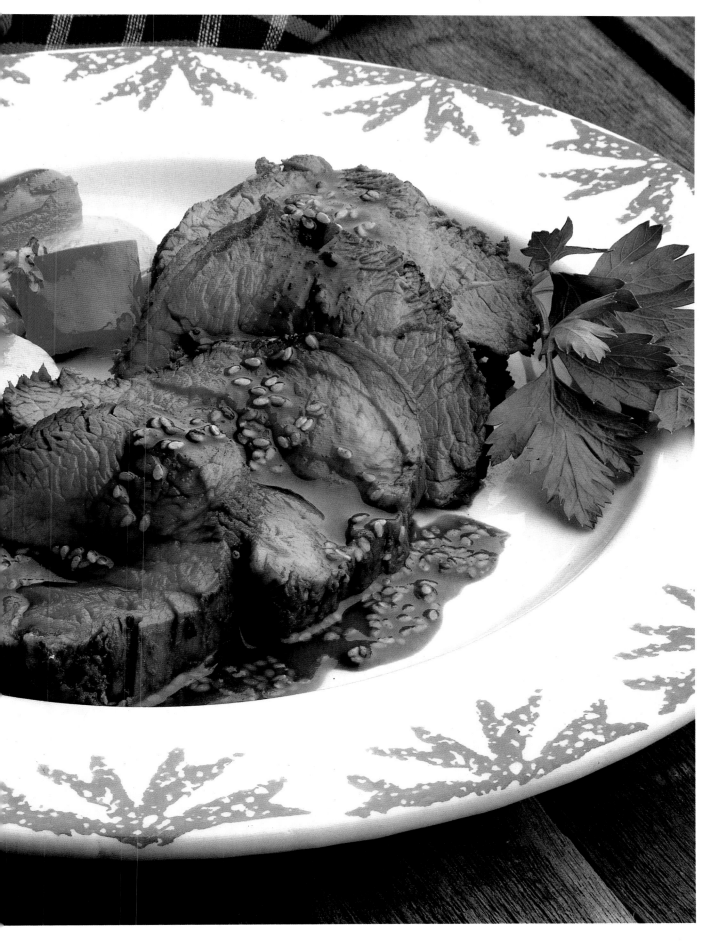

Veal with Tomato Mushroom Sauce

1382 kilojoules/330 calories per serving

1½ tblspn lite margarine

500g (1lb) veal fillet, cut into thin strips

1½ cups degreased chicken stock

½ cup white wine

2 tblspn tomato paste

1 tspn ground cumin

2 cups halved button mushrooms

1 tblspn Italian parsley

1 Melt the margarine in a large frying pan over moderate heat. Add the veal strips and cook, stirring constantly for 1 minute, remove with a slotted spoon and set aside.

2 Add the stock, wine, tomato paste, cumin and mushrooms to the frying pan, bring to the boil, reduce heat and simmer for 10 minutes.

3 Remove mushrooms with slotted spoon, set aside. Reduce pan liquid by half. Stir reserved veal strips and mushrooms into sauce, garnish with Italian parsley.

Serves 4

Minute Steak with Mushroom Wine Sauce

1130 kilojoules/270 calories per serving

8 minute steaks, 60g (2oz) each

1 tblspn unsalted butter

2 tspn olive oil

½ cup chopped onion

½ cup dry red wine

¼ cup chopped Italian parsley

1 cup thinly sliced button mushrooms

1 Flatten minute steaks between sheets of greaseproof paper.

2 Heat olive oil and butter in a large frying pan, add onion, saute until onion is golden, about 5 minutes.

3 Add steaks, wine and parsley, cook about 4 minutes, turning steaks once. Remove steaks to a heated platter, keep warm.

4 Add mushrooms to frying pan, saute until softened, about 4 minutes. Pour contents of pan over steaks. Serve immediately.

Serves 4

Saltimbocca

1151 kilojoules/275 calories per serving

4 veal scallopini, tenderised, 100g (3½oz) each

4 tblspn plain flour

1 tblspn lite margarine

4 slices lean ham, 50g (1¾oz) each

¾ cup grated mozzarella cheese

1 Lightly flour each veal scallopini. Melt margarine in a large frying pan over moderate heat, add veal, cook 30 seconds each side, remove from heat.

2 Place a slice of ham on top of each scallopini, top with mozzarella cheese. Bake in a moderately hot oven for 10 minutes, or until cheese has melted. Serve with a small salad if desired.

Serves 4

Marinated Loin of Veal

963 kilojoules/230 calories per serving

½ cup chopped fresh coriander leaves

750g (1½lb) loin of veal, boned

MARINADE

1 cup white wine

½ onion, roughly chopped

¼ cup white wine vinegar

1 clove garlic, halved

2 tspn freshly squeezed lemon juice

1 To make marinade: Combine wine, onion, vinegar, garlic and lemon juice in a processor, puree.

2 Spread coriander leaves all over veal, pressing well in with your hands. Place veal in a dish just large enough to hold it, pour over marinade. Cover, refrigerate overnight. Turn meat every couple of hours.

3 Allow meat to return to room temperature. Remove coriander leaves, reserve marinade. Place meat under a moderate pre-heated griller, cook for about 1 hour, or until tender. Baste with marinade and turn from time to time to allow for even cooking.

4 Allow veal to stand at room temperature for 10 minutes, before carving thinly.

Serves 6

Veal Scallopini with Herbed Lemon Sauce

1068 kilojoules/255 calories per serving

8 veal scallopini, 60g (2oz) each

LEMON SAUCE

⅔ cup freshly squeezed lemon juice

½ cup dry white wine

2 cloves garlic, crushed

2 tblspn olive oil

¼ cup finely chopped continental parsley

¼ cup finely chopped fresh basil

pepper

basil sprigs for garnish

1 To make Lemon Sauce: Combine lemon juice, wine, garlic, oil and herbs in a screwtop jar. Add freshly ground pepper to taste. Shake until well combined.

2 Brush scallopini with the lemon sauce.

3 Pre-heat the griller, place scallopini on griller tray, cook about 4 minutes, turning once, brushing with the sauce.

4 Place the veal in a heated serving dish, spoon over remaining sauce. Garnish with basil.

Serves 4

Top: Veal with Tomato Mushroom Sauce. Bottom: Saltimbocca

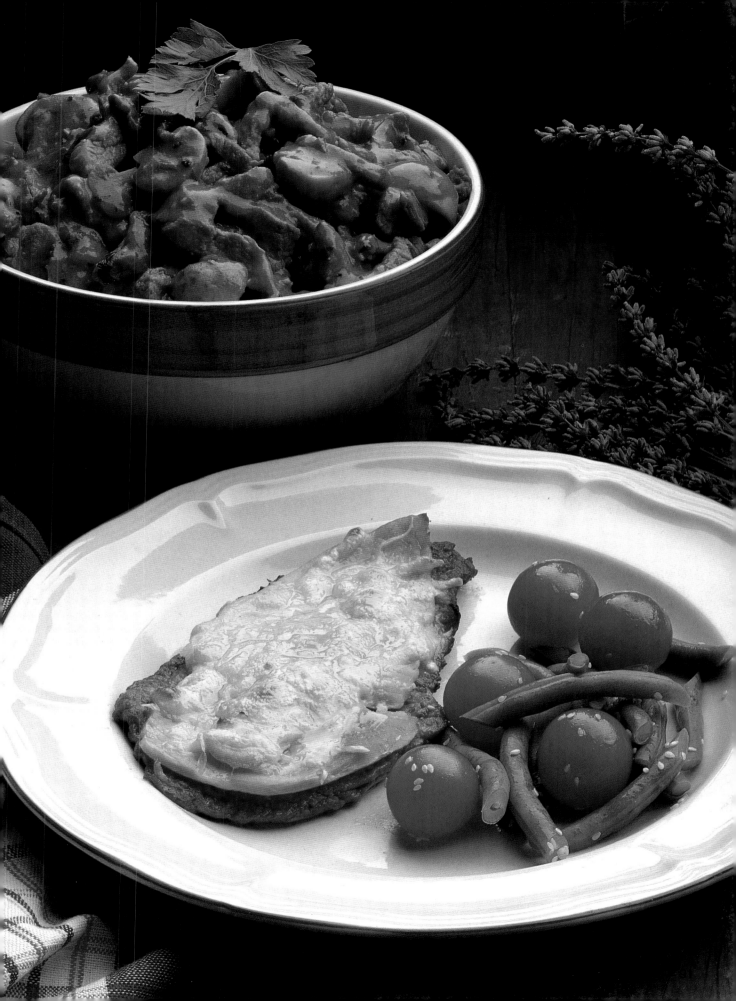

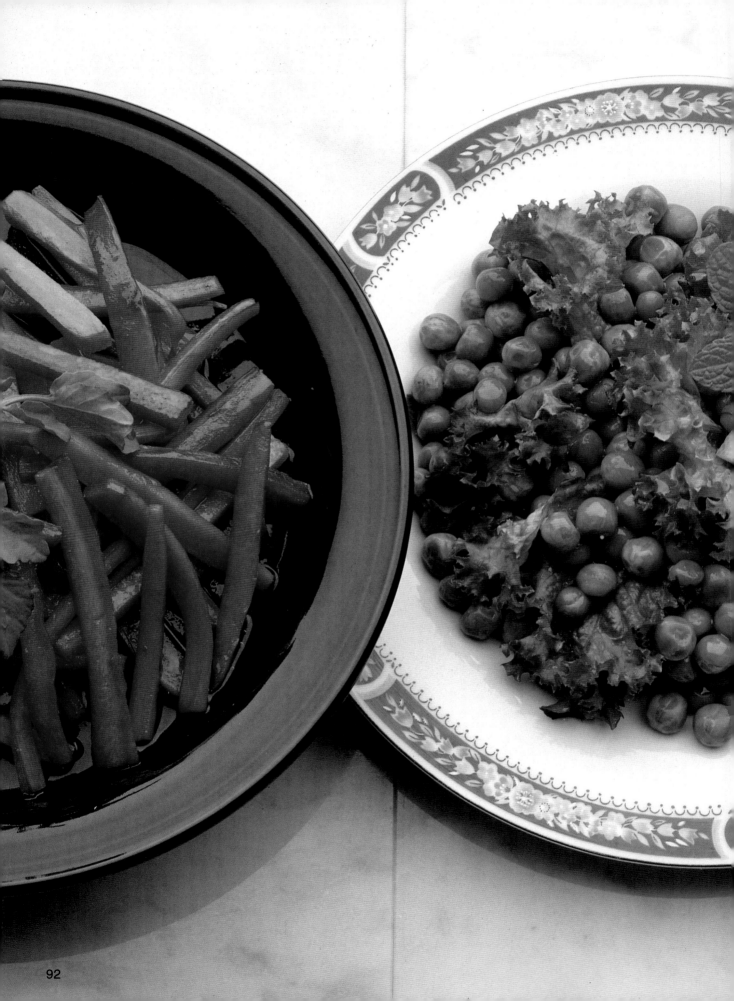

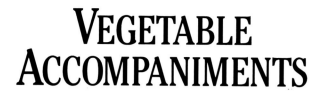

VEGETABLE ACCOMPANIMENTS

Vegetables are high in fibre, low in fat and packed full of vitamins. These mouthwatering recipes are perfect accompaniments to lean meat and fish.

Honey Glazed Carrot Straws

356 kilojoules/85 calories per serving

1 tblspn oil

1½ tblspn honey

2 tblspn red wine vinegar

6 medium carrots, peeled and cut into batons

watercress sprig for garnish

1 Heat the oil, honey and red wine vinegar in a medium frying pan over moderate heat until honey turns dark brown, about 3 minutes.

2 Add the carrots to the frying pan and toss in the honey glaze. Cook, stirring constantly, for 3 minutes or until carrots are just tender.

3 Serve immediately and garnish with watercress.

Serves 4

Mustard Coated Zucchini (Courgette)

335 kilojoules/80 calories per serving

500g (1lb) zucchini (courgette)

30g (1oz) unsalted butter, melted

1 tblspn whole grain mustard

1 Rinse zucchini thoroughly under cold running water. Cut in half lengthwise.

Far Left: Honey Glazed Carrot Straws. Left: Peas and Lettuce with Mint and Lemon

2 Brush zucchini on both sides with melted butter, place on a pre-heated griller tray, cut side down. Grill about 2 minutes.

3 Turn zucchini over, brush cut sides with mustard. Grill until golden and tender.

Serves 4

Peas and Lettuce with Mint and Lemon

293 kilojoules/70 calories per serving

1½ cups frozen peas, thawed

1 tblspn lite margarine

2 tspn freshly squeezed lemon juice

1 tspn julienned lemon rind

1 tblspn finely chopped fresh mint

1 curly endive or coral lettuce, washed and torn into pieces

4 lemon slices for garnish

1 Cook the peas in boiling water until just tender, drain well. Add the margarine to the peas and toss well.

2 Stir in the lemon juice, lemon rind and mint.

3 Arrange peas with the lettuce on each serving plate, garnish with lemon slices.

Serves 4

Broccoli and Pear Puree

502 kilojoules/120 calories per serving

560g (1lb 2oz) broccoli, stems and flowerets separated

3 tspn olive oil

2 tblspn finely chopped onion

1 firm pear, peeled, quartered, cored, thinly sliced

⅓ cup degreased chicken stock

1 tblspn cream

pinch nutmeg

salt

pepper

1 Peel broccoli stems, cut into 1cm (½in) pieces. Place in a steamer basket, together with flowerets. Steam until bright green and tender, about 12 minutes.

2 Heat oil in a frying pan, add onion, saute until soft, about 5 minutes. Add pear slices and chicken stock, bring to a boil.

3 Reduce heat, cook gently until pear is tender, about 4 minutes. Add broccoli, allow to heat through, transfer to a processor.

4 Add cream and nutmeg, puree until smooth. Season to taste with salt and freshly ground pepper. Serve immediately.

Serves 4

Potato and Leek Gratin

754 kilojoules/180 calories per serving

5 medium potatoes, peeled and sliced into thin rounds

1 cup chicken stock

2 large leeks, washed and sliced (white part only)

2 cloves garlic, crushed

1 tblspn finely chopped fresh rosemary

2 tblspn lite margarine

½ cup dried breadcrumbs

1 Bring a large saucepan of water to the boil, add the potato slices and cook for 7 minutes. Remove with a slotted spoon and refresh under cold water, set aside.

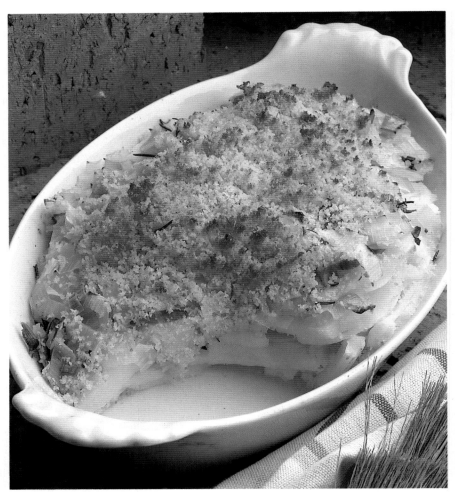

Potato and Leek Gratin

2 In a small saucepan, combine the stock, leeks, garlic and rosemary. Bring to the boil, lower the heat and simmer for 3 minutes.

3 Arrange the potato slices in layers in an ovenproof dish and top with the leek mixture.

4 Melt the margarine and stir in the breadcrumbs. Sprinkle over the top of the leek mixture and bake in a moderate oven for 25-30 minutes.

Serves 4

Foil Baked Potatoes with Dill

670 kilojoules/160 calories per serving

4 medium potatoes, scrubbed, not peeled

¼ cup unsalted butter, melted

2 tblspn chopped fresh dill

salt

pepper

1 Cut potatoes into ¼cm (⅛in) slices, but do not cut right through to the bottom.

2 Combine melted butter in a small bowl with dill, season with salt and freshly ground pepper.

3 Cut 4 pieces of foil, large enough to enfold potatoes comfortably. Brush foil with a little of the butter mixture in the centre.

4 Place a potato on top, spread the slices gently, brush with the butter mixture. Repeat with remaining potatoes.

5 Cook in a 180°C (350°F) oven until potatoes are tender, about 45 minutes, or cook on a barbecue. Open packages carefully to allow steam to escape. Serve hot.

Serves 4

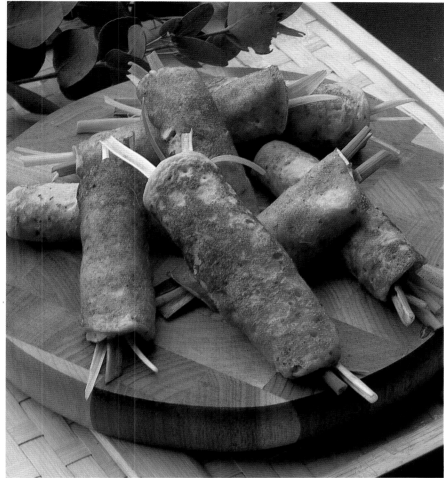

Red Capsicum (Pepper) Pancakes with Spring Onions (Scallions)

Capsicum (Pepper) Medley Stir-fry

293 kilojoules/70 calories per serving

1 tblspn olive oil

2 large cloves garlic, finely chopped

2 carrots, cut diagonally into ¼cm (⅛in) slices

½ green capsicum (pepper), cut into julienne strips

½ red capsicum (pepper), cut into julienne strips

½ yellow capsicum (pepper), cut into julienne strips

1 small Spanish onion, sliced, rings separated

1 cup thinly sliced button mushrooms

2 tblspn chopped fresh coriander

1 Heat oil in a frying pan, add garlic, saute until golden. Add carrot, saute 2 minutes.

2 Add green, red and yellow capsicum and onion, stir-fry 2 minutes.

3 Add mushrooms, stir-fry a further 2 minutes or until all vegetables are nearly tender, but still crisp. Sprinkle with coriander, toss to mix. Serve hot.

Serves 4

Red and Green Sauteed Potatoes

314 kilojoules/75 calories per serving

8 baby new potatoes, halved

1 tblspn unsalted butter

1 tblspn chopped spring onions (scallion)

1 tblspn chopped red capsicum (pepper)

1 tblspn chopped green capsicum (pepper)

salt

pepper

1 tblspn chopped parsley

1 Steam potatoes until tender, about 12 minutes.

2 Melt butter in a frying pan, add spring onion and red and green capsicum. Saute until heated through, about 2 minutes.

3 Add potato halves, saute 2 minutes or until potatoes turn golden. Transfer to a heated serving dish, season to taste with salt and freshly ground pepper. Scatter with parsley, serve hot.

Serves 4

Red Capsicum (Pepper) Pancakes with Spring Onions (Scallions)

502 kilojoules/120 calories per serving, 3 each

1 red capsicum (pepper), seeded and chopped

½ cup ricotta cheese

2 egg-whites

¼ cup flour

½ tspn cracked black pepper

½ onion, peeled and roughly chopped

8 spring onions (scallions), cut into big strips

1 In a blender or food processor, blend the red capsicum with ricotta cheese, egg-whites, flour, pepper and onion for about 2 minutes.

2 Heat a non-stick frying pan to moderate heat. Drop table-spoonfuls of batter into the frying pan. Cook until the underneath side is golden and the topside is just dry. Turn pancakes over and cook until other side browns.

3 Remove pancakes from heat, place a few strips of spring onions inside each pancake and roll up. Serve immediately.

Makes 12

Minted Honey Onions

502 kilojoules/120 calories per serving

2 tspn lite margarine

500g (1lb) baby onions, peeled and halved

2 tblspn honey

3 tblspn soy sauce

2 tblspn Worcestershire sauce

1 tblspn finely chopped mint

1 Melt margarine in a medium frying pan over moderate heat, add onions and toss gently.

2 Stir in the honey, soy sauce and Worcestershire sauce. Cover frying pan and cook over low heat for 10 minutes, stirring occasionally.

3 Stir in the mint and serve immediately.

Serves 4

Celery with Toasted Almonds

314 kilojoules/75 calories per serving

30g (1oz) slivered almonds

1½ cups degreased chicken stock

1½ cups water

1 onion, chopped

8 sprigs continental parsley

12 peppercorns

1 blade mace

18 stalks celery, cut diagonally into 4cm (1½in) pieces

½ red capsicum (pepper), cut into 0.5cm (¼in) dice

½ yellow capsicum (pepper), cut into 0.5cm (¼in) dice

1 Spread almonds on a baking tray, roast in a 180°C (350°F) oven for 10 minutes, or until golden. Set aside.

2 In a saucepan combine stock, water, onion, parsley, peppercorns and mace. Bring to a boil, reduce heat to moderately low, boil gently, uncovered, until liquid has been reduced to 1 cup, about 30 minutes. Strain.

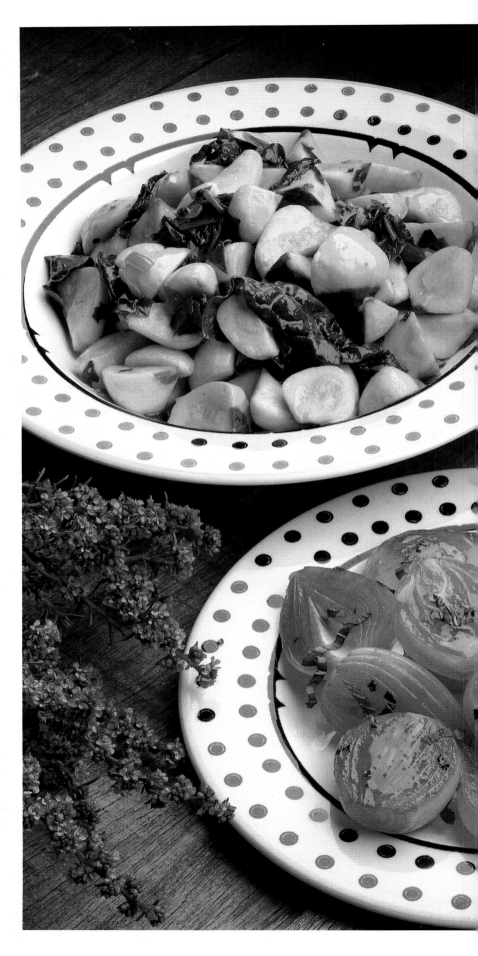

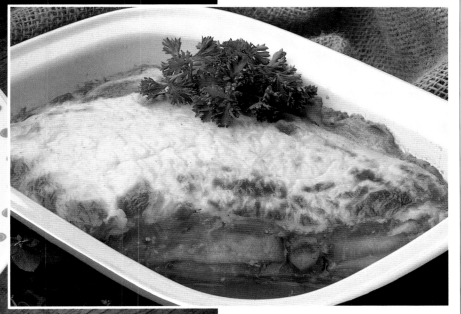

Left Top: Stir-fried Baby Squash and Spinach. Left Bottom: Minted Honey Onions. Below: Layered Eggplant (Aubergine) and Artichoke Bake

3 Add the spinach and cook for a further 1 minute. Serve vegetables immediately.

Serves 4

Layered Eggplant (Aubergine) and Artichoke Bake

1382 kilojoules/330 calories per serving

2 medium eggplants (aubergine), cut into thin slices

2 medium onions, sliced

1½ cups tinned tomatoes

2 cloves garlic

2 tspn mixed herbs

1 cup artichoke hearts, roughly chopped

2 medium tomatoes, sliced

100g (3½oz) cottage cheese

50g (1¾oz) ricotta cheese

½ cup grated mature cheese

1 egg-white

¼ cup skim milk

parsley sprig, for garnish

1 Place ½ cup of water in a large frying pan over moderate heat. Add the eggplant slices and cook for 3 minutes. Remove with a slotted spoon and place on absorbent paper, discard water.

2 Return frying pan to heat, add onions, tinned tomatoes, garlic and herbs, simmer for 5-7 minutes or until sauce thickens, stir in artichoke hearts.

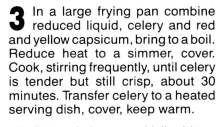

3 In a large frying pan combine reduced liquid, celery and red and yellow capsicum, bring to a boil. Reduce heat to a simmer, cover. Cook, stirring frequently, until celery is tender but still crisp, about 30 minutes. Transfer celery to a heated serving dish, cover, keep warm.

4 Return frying pan with liquid to a high heat, boil until reduced to 3 tablespoons. Pour over celery, sprinkle with almonds. Serve immediately.

Serves 8

Stir-fried Baby Squash and Spinach

272 kilojoules/65 calories per serving

8 spinach leaves, torn into bite-size pieces

1 tblspn oil

2 tblspn tarragon vinegar

2 cups baby yellow squash, cut into quarters

1 Bring a medium saucepan of water to the boil. Add the spinach and cook for 1 minute, refresh under cold water and set aside.

2 Heat the oil and vinegar in a large frying pan. Add the squash and cook, stirring constantly, for 2 minutes.

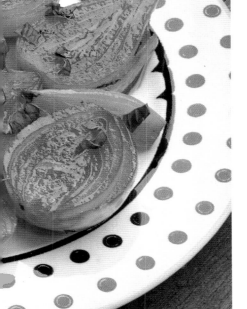

3 Place half the tomato slices over the bottom of an ovenproof baking dish. Top with half the eggplant slices, then pour half the tomato mixture over the top. Repeat with remaining tomato slices, eggplant slices and tomato mixture.

4 In a food processor or blender, process the cottage cheese, ricotta cheese, mature cheese, egg-white and skim milk until smooth. Spread mixture over the top and bake in a moderate oven for 30 minutes.

Serves 4

PASTA AND EGGS

Pasta is rich in complex carbohydrate and contains no fat. Eggs are a good source of protein, vitamins and minerals. As such these two foods are nutritious and excellent for a low kilojoule diet.

Baked Spanish Omelette

1005 kilojoules/240 calories per serving

625g (1lb 4oz) potatoes, peeled and cut into cubes

250g (½lb) leeks, thoroughly rinsed, thinly sliced

250g (½lb) cauliflowerets

2 zucchini (courgette), thinly sliced

2 small red capsicum (peppers), seeded, cut into thin strips

8 eggs

1¾ cups skim milk

1 tblspn finely chopped parsley

1 tspn paprika

2 cloves garlic, crushed

salt

pepper

4 large tomatoes, thinly sliced

4 tblspn grated low fat Cheddar cheese

1 Cook potatoes in boiling salted water for 10 minutes. Drain well. Place in a lightly oiled round baking dish. Cover with slices of leek, cauliflowerets, zucchini slices and capsicum strips.

2 Mix together eggs, milk, parsley, paprika and garlic, season to taste with salt and freshly ground pepper. Pour over vegetables. Cover with tomato slices and grated cheese. Bake in a moderate oven for 45 minutes or until golden brown on top. Allow to stand at room temperature for 5 minutes before serving.

Serves 8

Fettucine with Red Capsicum (Pepper) and Goat's Cheese

1089 kilojoules/260 calories per serving

410g (13oz) dried fettucine

2 tblspn oil

2 cloves garlic, crushed

2 red capsicum (pepper), seeded and cut into small strips

8 spring onions (scallions), cut into thin strips

1 tspn cracked black pepper

100g (3½oz) goat's cheese, crumbled into small pieces

1 Bring a large saucepan of water to the boil, add the fettucine and cook until just tender.

2 Meanwhile, heat the oil over medium heat, add the garlic and red capsicum, cook for 2 minutes. Add the spring onions and pepper and cook for a further 1 minute.

3 Drain pasta and add to the red capsicum mixture, toss well. Carefully stir in the cheese and divide pasta between 4 serving dishes. Serve immediately.

Serves 4

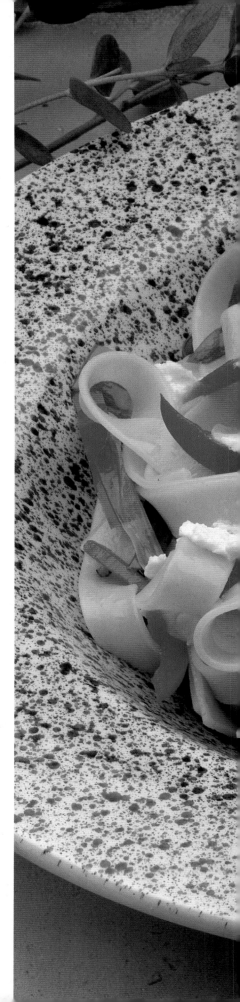

Fettucine with Red Capsicum (Pepper) and Goat's Cheese

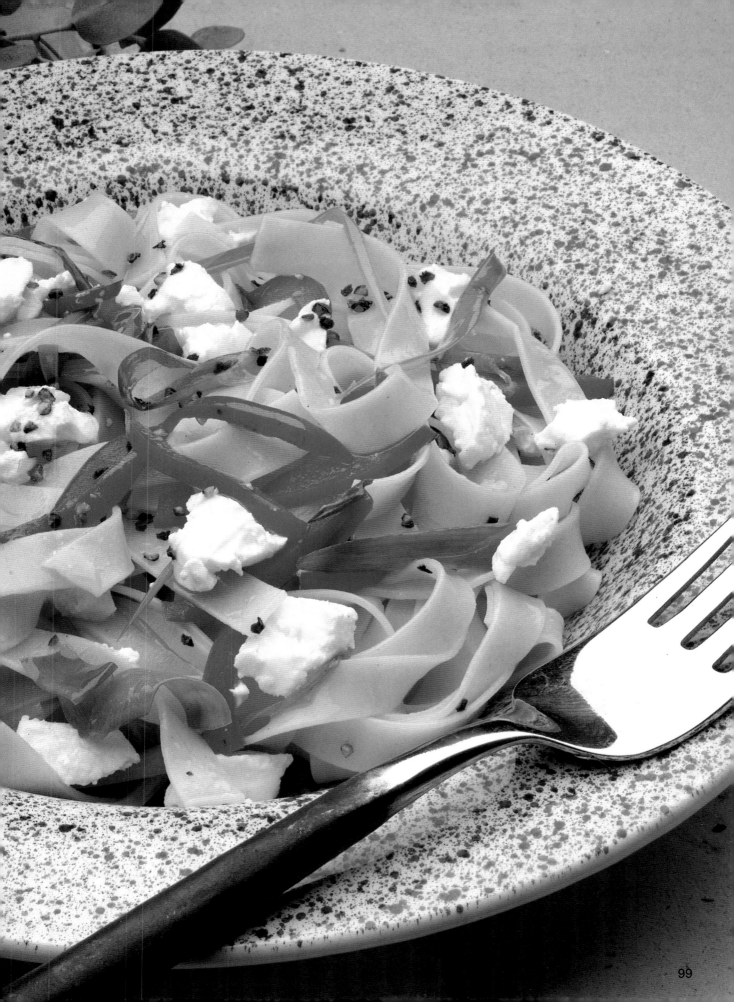

Mediterranean Buckwheat Pancakes

1005 kilojoules/240 calories per serving

PANCAKES

1 egg

300ml (½ pint) skim milk

1 tspn sunflower oil

60g (2oz) wholemeal flour

60g (2oz) buckwheat flour

FILLING

2 tspn olive oil

1 onion, thinly sliced

1 clove garlic, crushed

1 eggplant (aubergine), unpeeled and cut into cubes

250g (½lb) zucchini (courgette), thinly sliced

250g (½lb) red and green capsicum (pepper), seeded and chopped

250g (½lb) tomatoes, chopped

3 tblspn tomato puree

1 tblspn chopped parsley

8 basil leaves, cut into strips

1 bay leaf

1 carton low fat plain yoghurt

1 tblspn chopped fresh parsley, extra

1 To make pancakes: Place egg, milk and oil in a blender. Liquidize for 30 seconds. Add flour, blend 1 minute. Set aside for 30 minutes.

2 Heat a little oil in a pancake pan. Wipe over with absorbent paper. Pour in 2 tablespoons of the batter and tilt until batter coats the bottom. Cook 2 minutes, toss and cook one minute on the other side, slide out of pan, keep warm. Place a piece of greaseproof paper between each pancake.

3 To make filling: Heat oil in a heavy pan. Fry onion and garlic for 5 minutes. Add eggplant, zucchini and capsicum, cook for 5 minutes. Add tomatoes, tomato puree, parsley, basil and bay leaf, bring to a boil. Reduce heat to a simmer and cook 15 minutes.

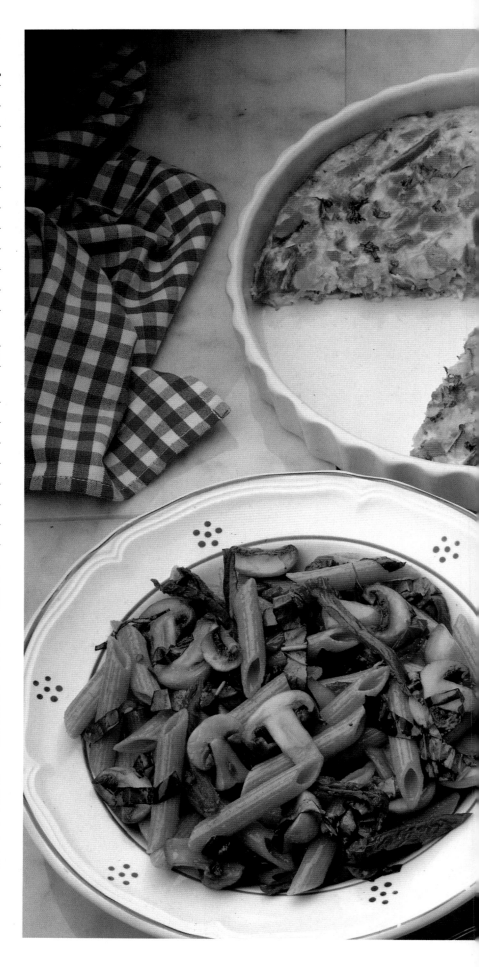

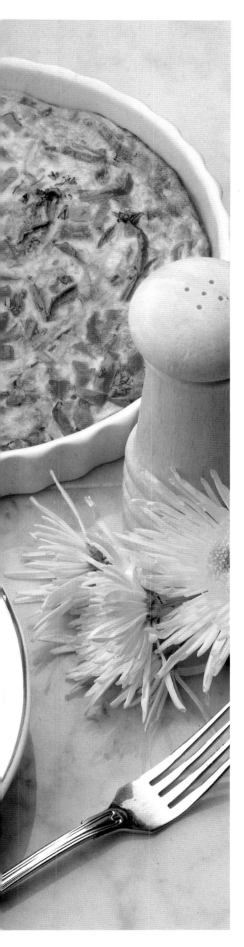

4 Place 2 tablespoons of the filling in each pancake. Roll up and place in a lightly oiled ovenproof serving dish. Cover with foil and place in a pre-heated oven for 15 minutes. Serve with a dollop of yoghurt and sprinkle with parsley.

Serves 8

Wholemeal Pasta with Mushrooms and Sun-dried Tomatoes

1151 kilojoules/275 calories per serving

410g (13oz) wholemeal macaroni

1 tblspn olive oil

2 cloves garlic, crushed

1 cup button mushrooms

¼ cup sun-dried tomatoes, cut into strips

2 tblspn chopped fresh basil

1 Bring a large saucepan of water to the boil, add the pasta and cook until just tender, drain.

2 Heat the oil in a large frying pan over moderate heat. Add the garlic, mushrooms and sun-dried tomatoes and cook for 2 minutes.

3 Stir in the basil and pasta, serve immediately.

Serves 4

Piperade

670 kilojoules/160 calories per serving

1 tblspn olive oil

2 green capsicum (pepper), seeded and cut into short strips

2 medium leeks, white part only, finely chopped

1 medium onion, finely chopped

2 ripe tomatoes, cut into small pieces

150g (5oz) lean leg ham, chopped

¼ cup chopped parsley

2 eggs

2 egg-whites

½ cup skim milk

Top: Piperade. Bottom: Wholemeal Pasta with Mushrooms and Sun-dried Tomatoes

1 Heat the oil in a large frying pan over medium heat. Add the capsicum, leeks and onion, cook for 3 minutes.

2 Add the tomatoes and ham and cook for a further 5 minutes, stir in the parsley and remove from heat.

3 Beat the eggs, egg-whites and milk together and pour into vegetable mixture, mix well.

4 Pour mixture into a greased 23cm (8in) ovenproof flan dish and bake in a moderate oven for 30 minutes or until cooked through, serve immediately.

Serves 6

Fettucine with Broad Beans, Red Capsicum (Pepper) and Grainy Mustard

1465 kilojoules/350 calories per serving

500g (1lb) red capsicum (pepper)

1½ cups degreased chicken stock

315g (10oz) broad beans

salt

pepper

1 onion, chopped

3 tblspn grainy mustard

2½ tblspn unsalted butter

500g (1lb) thin fettucine

1 Char capsicum over a gas flame or under a griller until blackened on all sides. Place in a paper bag and allow to stand 10 minutes to steam. Peel and seed capsicum, cut into 0.5cm (¼in) wide strips. Set aside.

2 Heat stock in a heavy pan over medium heat and bring to a simmer. Add broad beans, season with salt and pepper to taste, cook 6 minutes. Add onion and grainy mustard, simmer one minute. Add butter and red capsicum strips. Stir gently and simmer 2 minutes.

3 Meanwhile, cook fettucine in boiling salted water for 8-10 minutes or until al dente. Drain and transfer to pan with broad bean mixture. Toss well and serve immediately.

Serves 8

Mushroom Lasagne

1633 kilojoules/390 calories per serving

30g (1oz) porcini mushrooms (see note)

2 tspn olive oil

2 onions, thinly sliced

2 cloves garlic, crushed

½ cup chopped Italian flat leaf parsley

500g (1lb) fresh mushrooms, sliced

2 tblspn cornflour

600ml (1 pint) skim milk

600ml (1 pint) low fat yoghurt

salt

pepper

750g (1½lb) broccoli flowerets

185g (6oz) celery, chopped

8 lasagne sheets

2 tspn cornflour, extra

3 tblspn freshly grated Parmesan cheese

1 Soak porcini in very hot water for 20-30 minutes. Drain through a fine sieve. Rinse thoroughly to remove any remaining grit. Pat dry with paper towels. Chop coarsely and set aside.

2 Heat oil in a heavy pan. Fry onion and garlic until soft. Add parsley and fresh mushrooms, cook 5 minutes.

3 Dissolve the cornflour in a little of the milk. Pour remaining milk over mushrooms and when heated through, stir in dissolved cornflour and cook, stirring continuously, for 5 minutes, or until sauce thickens. Remove from heat, stir in porcini, 300ml (½ pint) of the yoghurt, season to taste with salt and freshly ground pepper.

4 Steam broccoli and celery for 5-6 minutes.

5 Cook lasagne in boiling salted water for 8-10 minutes, or until al dente. Put a layer of mushroom sauce into the bottom of an ovenproof serving dish. Cover with a layer of lasagne, then the broccoli and celery, then the mushroom sauce. Repeat, making sure to end with lasagne.

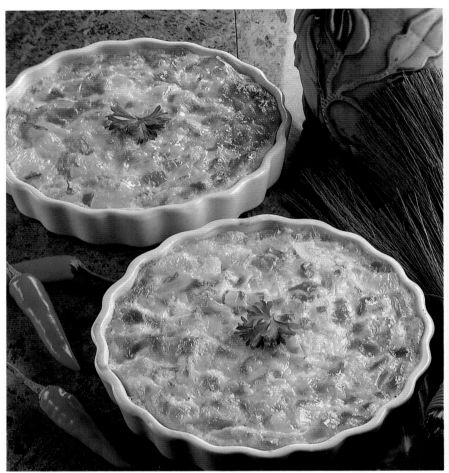

Individual Ham and Pineapple Frittatas

6 Mix 2 teaspoons cornflour with remaining yoghurt. Pour over lasagne. Sprinkle with Parmesan cheese and bake in a moderate oven for 25-30 minutes. Serve hot.

Note: Porcini are dried Italian mushrooms with a marvellous flavour. They are available in delicatessens and Italian groceries.

Serves 8

Avocado Frittata

984 kilojoules/235 calories per serving

½ avocado, cut into 1cm (½in) cubes

1 tspn freshly squeezed lemon juice

½ tspn salt

30g (1oz) cream cheese

1 tblspn finely chopped chives

6 olives, stoned and thinly sliced

6 eggs

pepper

2 tspn olive oil

1 Toss avocado in lemon juice and salt. Add cream cheese in small spoonfuls. Add chives and olives. Toss gently.

2 Beat eggs with freshly ground pepper to taste. Heat oil in a heavy omelette pan, add eggs and cook about 2 minutes, or until bottom is set. Remove from heat and gently spread avocado mixture over top of frittata.

3 Place frittata under a griller, about 10cm (4in) from heat, cook about 2 minutes, until edges are brown and frittata is set. Serve immediately.

Serves 6

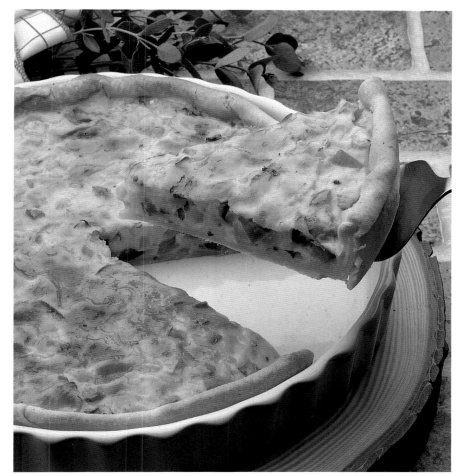

Celery and Green Capsicum (Pepper) Flan

Celery and Green Capsicum (Pepper) Flan

921 kilojoules/220 calories per serving

1 sheet ready-rolled shortcrust pastry

1¾ cups skim milk

1 onion, peeled and chopped

1 tblspn oil

6 stalks celery, chopped

1 green capsicum (pepper), seeded and chopped

2 tblspn finely chopped spring onions (scallions)

1½ tblspn plain flour

1 egg

2 egg-whites

½ tspn cracked black pepper

1 Roll out sheet of pastry to fit a greased 20cm (8in) ovenproof flan dish, bake blind for 10 minutes in a moderately hot oven.

2 To make filling: Heat the milk in a medium saucepan over moderate heat. Add the onion and bring to the boil. Strain the milk and set aside.

3 Heat the oil in a large saucepan over low heat, add the celery, capsicum and spring onions and cook for 5 minutes.

4 Add the flour and cook for 1 minute, stirring constantly. Pour the reserved milk into the flour, mix well and bring sauce to the boil, remove from heat.

5 Cool sauce to room temperature, beat in the eggs, egg-whites and pepper.

6 Pour mixture into pastry case and cook for 35 minutes in a moderate oven.

Serves 6

Individual Ham and Pineapple Frittatas

628 kilojoules/150 calories per serving

1 tblspn lite margarine

1 onion, peeled and chopped

1 clove garlic, crushed

½ cup lean ham, chopped

¼ tspn finely chopped fresh chilli

1 red capsicum (pepper), seeded and finely chopped

2 spring onions (scallions), chopped

¾ cup tinned unsweetened pineapple pieces, drained

1 tblspn finely chopped fresh parsley

2 eggs

2 egg-whites

¾ cup skim milk

¼ cup grated mature cheese

1 Heat the margarine in a large frying pan over moderate heat. Add the onion, garlic, ham, chilli, red capsicum and spring onions and cook for 3 minutes.

2 Stir in the pineapple pieces and parsley, remove from heat and cool to room temperature.

3 Whisk together the eggs, milk and cheese and mix into ham and pineapple mixture.

4 Pour mixture into 4 individual 10-12cm (4-5in) greased oven-proof flan dishes, bake in moderate oven for 20-25 minutes.

Serves 4

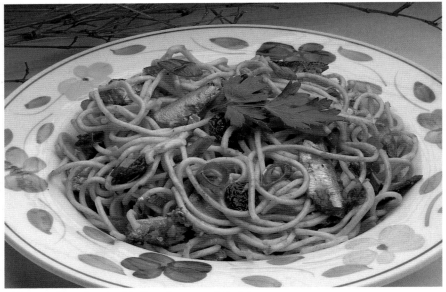

Above: Spaghetti with Sardines and Raisins

Parsnip and Butter Bean Crepes

1340 kilojoules/320 calories per serving

CREPES

¾ cup plain flour

3 eggs, lightly beaten

1 tblspn water

1 cup skim milk

FILLING

1 cup cooked parsnip

1 cup butter beans, drained

½ cup ricotta cheese

1 clove garlic, crushed

2 tblspn freshly squeezed lemon juice

2 tblspn chopped parsley

SAUCE

¾ cup tomato puree

2 tblspn dry white wine

¼ tspn ground black pepper

1 Sift flour into a medium bowl, make a well in the centre, add the combined eggs, water and milk, gradually whisk the liquid into flour until batter is smooth. Strain batter if there are any lumps.

2 Heat the crepe pan over medium heat, brush lightly with oil. Pour 3-4 tablespoons of batter evenly into the pan, cook crepe until golden, turn with spatula and cook until light and golden on underside.

3 To make filling: Combine parsnip, beans, ricotta cheese, garlic, lemon juice and parsley with a fork, mash well. Spread filling inside each crepe and fold up.

4 To make sauce: Combine tomato puree with the white wine and pepper in a medium saucepan over moderate heat, until sauce is hot. Serve with crepes.

Makes 10-12
Serves 3

Crunchy Macaroni Cheese

1507 kilojoules/360 calories per serving

185g (6oz) macaroni (see note)

½ onion

1 sprig thyme

300ml (½ pint) skim milk

2 tblspn unsalted butter

1½ tblspn plain flour (see note)

2 tblspn finely chopped chives

salt

pepper

1 fennel bulb, roughly chopped

60g (2oz) grated mature cheese

1 Cook macaroni in boiling salted water until al dente. Drain.

Right: Parsnip and Butter Bean Crepes

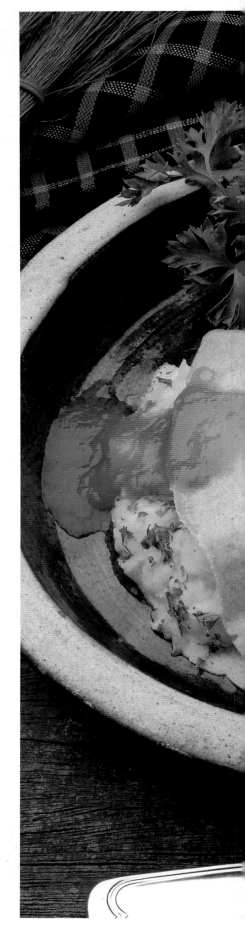

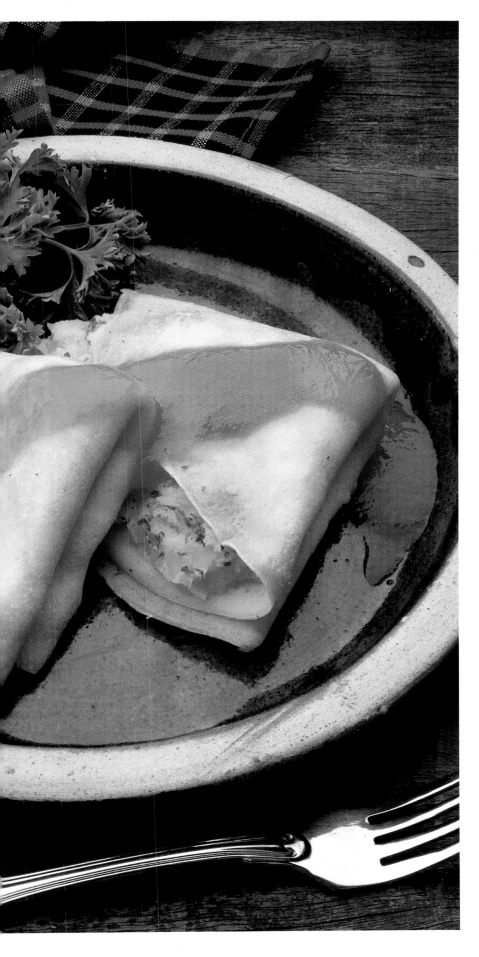

2 Combine onion, thyme and milk in a saucepan, bring to a boil. Remove pan from heat, allow to stand for 10 minutes. Remove onion and thyme.

3 In another saucepan melt butter over gentle heat, stir in flour, cook for 5 minutes, stirring constantly. Remove from heat, add milk all at once, stirring vigorously.

4 Return to the heat, bring to a boil. Cook until sauce thickens, stirring constantly. Season with chives and salt and freshly ground pepper to taste.

5 Add macaroni and chopped fennel, cook 2 minutes. Spoon into an ovenproof serving dish, sprinkle with cheese.

6 Bake in 190°C (375°F) oven until top is golden, about 30 minutes. Serve hot.

Note: To further increase the goodness of this dish, use wholemeal macaroni and flour.

Serves 4

Spaghetti with Sardines and Raisins

1507 kilojoules/360 calories per serving

410g (13oz) spaghetti

1 tblspn olive oil

1 clove garlic, crushed

2 spring onions (scallions), sliced

2 tblspn raisins

2 x 110g (3½oz) cans sardines in tomato sauce

1 Bring a large saucepan of water to the boil, add the spaghetti and cook until just tender, drain.

2 Heat the oil in a medium saucepan over moderate heat. Add the garlic, spring onions and raisins, cook for 2 minutes.

3 Stir in the sardines and spaghetti, toss well and serve immediately.

Serves 4

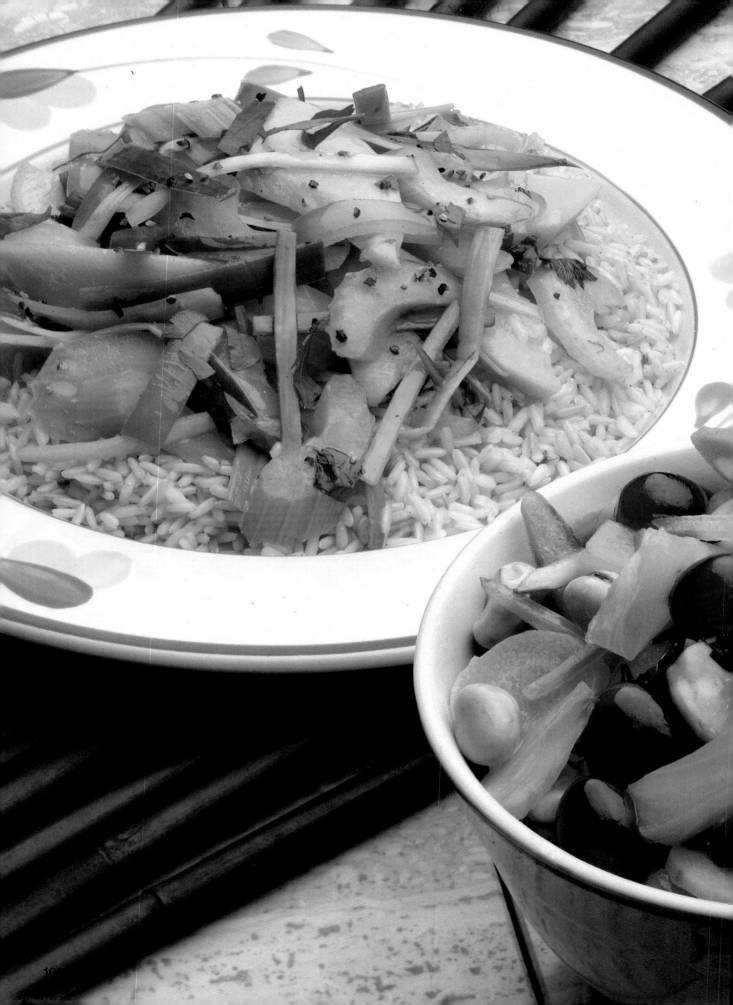

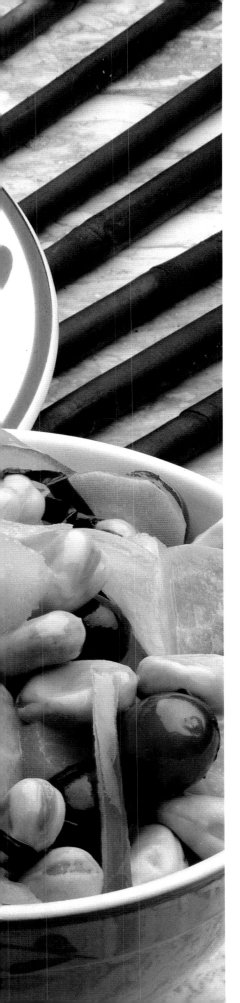

BEANS, PULSES AND RICE

Legumes are an important part of a nutritious diet because they are low in fat but high in protein and B group vitamins. They contribute important dietary fibre.

Pawpaw (Papaya) Vegetable Stir-fry and Rice

523 kilojoules/125 calories per serving

1 cup brown rice

1 tblspn oil

3 tblspn red wine vinegar

2 stalks celery, sliced

1 red onion, peeled and sliced

1 leek, cut into thin strips

¼ tspn cracked black pepper

½ pawpaw (papaya), seeded, peeled and sliced

1 tblspn chopped Italian parsley

1 Bring a large saucepan of water to the boil, add the rice and cook until just tender, about 25 minutes.

2 Heat the oil in a large frying pan or wok. When the oil is hot, add the vinegar, celery, onion, leek and pepper and cook, stirring constantly, for 2-3 minutes.

3 Stir in the pawpaw and parsley and cook for a further 1 minute. Serve stir-fry over the rice.

Serves 4

Fruity Bean Stir-fry

879 kilojoules/210 calories per serving

315g (10oz) broad beans

1 tblspn oil

1 red onion, peeled and sliced

2 medium carrots, peeled and sliced

1 cup apple cider

1 tblspn chopped fresh basil

½ cup tinned unsweetened pineapple slices, drained

¾ cup black grapes

1 Bring a medium saucepan of water to the boil, add the beans, cook for 7 minutes, drain and set aside.

2 Heat the oil in a large frying pan or wok, add the onion and cook for 2 minutes. Add the carrots, cider and basil, cook for 3 minutes.

3 Stir in the pineapple and grapes and cook for a further 2 minutes. Serve hot or cold.

Serves 4

Top: Pawpaw (Papaya) Vegetable Stir-fry and Rice. Bottom: Fruity Bean Stir-fry

Oven-baked Tomatoes with Cannellini Stuffing

1047 kilojoules/250 calories per serving

125g (4oz) cannellini beans, soaked overnight

4 large, firm tomatoes

pepper

4 spring onions (scallions), finely chopped

2 cloves garlic, very finely chopped

2 tspn olive oil

250g (½lb) tomatoes, peeled, chopped

1½ tblspn tomato puree

12 black olives, coarsely chopped

2 tblspn chopped fresh parsley

salt

½ firm avocado, peeled, cut into 0.5cm (¼in) cubes

60g (2oz) mozzarella cheese, coarsely grated

1 Drain beans, place in a saucepan with plenty of water to cover, bring to a boil, reduce heat to a steady simmer, cook until tender, about 30-60 minutes, depending on age of beans. Drain.

2 Cut slice off rounded side of tomato, opposite stalk end, scoop out flesh and seeds. Season inside with freshly ground pepper, leave to drain upside down.

3 In a casserole, combine spring onion, garlic and oil. Saute gently until softened, about 3 minutes. Add tomatoes, tomato puree, olives and parsley, season to taste with salt. Cover, cook gently for 20 minutes, stirring from time to time.

4 Add beans and avocado, mix in gently. Season to taste with freshly ground pepper. Spoon mixture into prepared tomato shells, sprinkle with grated mozzarella.

5 Place filled tomatoes in an ovenproof serving dish, pour ¼ cup water into dish. Cover, bake in a 180°C (350°F) oven for 30 minutes, or until tomatoes and filling are heated through and cheese is bubbly. Serve hot.

Serves 4

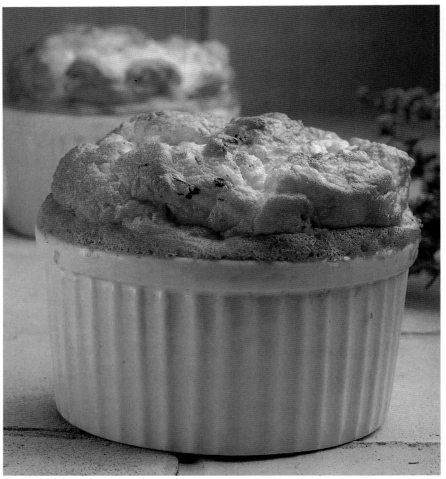

Broccoli and Rice Souffle

Broccoli and Rice Souffle

1130 kilojoules/270 calories per serving

1 tblspn butter

½ medium onion, peeled and finely chopped

2 tblspn plain flour

1 cup skim milk, heated

pinch salt

pinch pepper

¼ tspn ground nutmeg

½ cup grated cheese

1 cup cooked rice

1 cup blanched broccoli flowerets

3 eggs, separated

1 In a small saucepan, heat the butter over medium heat until bubbly, add onion and saute for 2 minutes. Reduce heat to low, add the flour and cook, stirring constantly, for 2 minutes.

2 Gradually whisk in the hot milk, add the salt, pepper and nutmeg. Stir until sauce thickens. Remove from the heat. Add the cheese, rice, broccoli and egg yolks, mix well.

3 In a large bowl, beat egg-whites until soft peaks form. Fold ¼ of the beaten egg-whites into broccoli mixture, then fold in the remaining whites.

4 Lightly grease four ¾-cup capacity souffle dishes and divide mixture between each dish. Bake in a moderate oven for 25 minutes. Serve immediately.

Serves 4

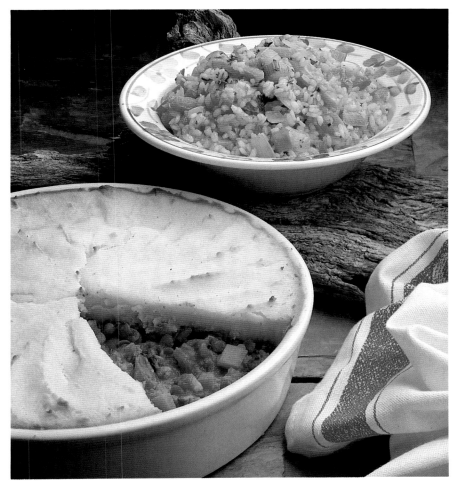

Top: Risotto Primavera. Bottom: Lentil and Vegetable Cottage Pie

Risotto Primavera

837 kilojoules/200 calories per serving

1 tblspn lite margarine

2 cloves garlic, crushed

1 onion, peeled and chopped

1 red capsicum (pepper), seeded and chopped

2 carrots, peeled and cut into thin strips

1½ cups Italian tomatoes with juice

1 tblspn chopped fresh parsley

2 cups short-grain rice

¼ tspn turmeric

2 celery sticks, chopped

3 cups water

2 tspn chopped fresh parsley, extra

1 Heat the margarine in a large frying pan over moderate heat. Add the garlic, onion, red capsicum and carrots, cook for 1 minute. Add the tomatoes and parsley and cook for a further 2 minutes.

2 Sprinkle the rice over the vegetables and stir for 1 minute. Add the turmeric, celery and water, cook, stirring occasionally, until water is absorbed and rice is cooked.

3 Sprinkle risotto with extra parsley to serve.

Serves 4

Curried Rice with Almonds

523 kilojoules/125 calories per serving

2 tspn unsalted butter

1 tblspn chopped onion

2 tblspn chopped celery

½ cup basmati rice

1 tblspn slivered almonds

½ tspn mild curry powder

1 Heat butter in a heavy-based saucepan, add onion and celery, saute until onion is golden, about 5 minutes.

2 Stir in rice, almonds and curry powder, cook until rice and almonds are lightly browned.

3 Add 1 cup hot water, mix well, bring to a boil. Reduce heat to a simmer, cover, cook until rice is tender and all liquid has been absorbed.

4 Fluff rice with a fork, serve hot.

Serves 4

Lentil and Vegetable Cottage Pie

1235 kilojoules/295 calories per serving

250g (½lb) brown lentils

2 bay leaves

1 tblspn oil

1 onion, peeled and chopped

4 carrots, peeled and chopped

2 celery sticks, chopped

1 tspn dried mixed herbs

1 tblspn chopped fresh parsley

1 cup tomato puree

¾ cup tinned tomatoes

1½ cups cooked potato, cut into cubes

3 tblspn skim milk

2 tblspn lite margarine

1 Wash the lentils, cover with fresh cold water and soak for 30 minutes. Drain and pour into a medium saucepan.

2 Cover with water, add bay leaves and bring to the boil over moderate heat. Reduce heat and simmer for 25 minutes. Drain lentils, remove bay leaves and set aside.

3 Heat the oil in a large frying pan over moderate heat. Add the onion, carrots and celery and cook for 4 minutes.

4 Add the lentils, herbs, parsley, tomato puree and tomatoes. Cover and simmer for 15 minutes. Pour the lentil mixture into the base of a large ovenproof dish.

5 Mash the potato with skim milk and margarine and spread on top of lentil mixture, bake in a moderate oven for 30 minutes.

Serves 6

Chickpea and Fresh Vegetable Casserole with Garlic Dill Dressing

691 kilojoules/165 calories per serving

125g (4oz) chickpeas, soaked overnight

1 cup broccoli flowerets

2 medium carrots, thinly sliced

2 tblspn chopped dill

60g (2oz) French beans, topped and tailed

1 medium red capsicum (pepper), cut into strips

150ml (¼ pint) boiling water

DRESSING

3 tblspn plain yoghurt

1 tblspn mayonnaise

2 tblspn chopped fresh dill

1 clove garlic, crushed

1 Drain chickpeas, place in a saucepan with plenty of fresh water to cover, bring to a boil, reduce heat to a simmer. Cook until chickpeas are tender, about 1-1½ hours, depending on age of chickpeas. Drain.

2 To make the dressing: Combine yoghurt, mayonnaise, dill and garlic in a small bowl. Stir until smooth. Cover, stand at room temperature for 20 minutes.

3 Place chickpeas in a casserole. Cover with broccoli and carrots, sprinkle with dill. Make a layer with the French beans and capsicum. Pour in boiling water, cover, bake in 180°C (350°F) oven for 15 minutes.

4 Pour over dressing, serve immediately. If desired, this casserole can be eaten at room temperature or chilled. In this case do not add dressing until ready to serve.

Serves 4

Spring Onion (Scallion) and Lemon Rice

586 kilojoules/140 calories per serving

1 tblspn olive oil

1 cup long-grain rice

2 cups chopped spring onions (scallion)

1 clove garlic, finely chopped

1¾ cups degreased chicken stock

2 tblspn freshly squeezed lemon juice

¼ cup chopped fresh coriander

1 tblspn sugar

salt

pepper

1 thinly sliced lemon

sprigs of fresh coriander for garnish

1 In a flameproof casserole, combine rice and oil. Saute over medium heat until rice is well coated and golden, about 5 minutes.

2 Add spring onion and garlic, saute until softened, about 3 minutes. Add chicken stock, lemon juice, coriander and sugar, season to taste with salt and freshly ground pepper.

3 Bring to a boil, reduce heat to a simmer, place lemon slices on top of rice. Cover, cook until rice is tender and all the liquid has been absorbed, about 20 minutes. Allow to stand off the heat for 10 minutes, without removing the lid. Serve hot, garnished with coriander sprigs.

Serves 8

Wild Rice and Mushroom Salad

607 kilojoules/145 calories per serving

1½ tblspn lite margarine

4 spring onions (scallions), chopped

1 leek, white part only, sliced

125g (4oz) button mushrooms, halved

1 cup wild rice, washed and drained

2½ cups chicken stock

1 Melt the margarine in a large frying pan over moderate heat. Add the spring onions, leek and mushrooms; cook for 3 minutes; remove with a slotted spoon and set aside.

2 Add the rice to the frying pan, stir to coat with the margarine. Add the stock and bring to the boil, reduce heat, simmer for 30 to 40 minutes, until rice is cooked and liquid is absorbed.

3 Stir in reserved spring onions, leeks and mushrooms before serving.

Serves 4

Fennel and Almond Risotto

1319 kilojoules/315 calories per serving

1 onion, chopped

2 tspn olive oil

500g (1lb) fennel, sliced

250g (½lb) Arborio rice

2 tblspn freshly squeezed lemon juice

60g (2oz) slivered almonds

375g (¾lb) tomatoes, peeled, seeded, chopped

salt

pepper

1 Combine onion and oil in a flameproof casserole, saute until onion is golden, about 5 minutes. Add fennel, cook 2 minutes.

2 Stir in rice, add 1 cup boiling water. Stir to mix, bring to a boil, cover, reduce heat to a simmer. Cook until all the liquid has been absorbed, stirring from time to time.

3 Add lemon juice, almonds, tomatoes and ½ cup boiling water. Stir well, cook until all liquid has been absorbed. If rice is not cooked by this stage, add a little more boiling water.

4 Season to taste with salt and freshly ground pepper, serve hot.

Serves 4

Polenta with Mushroom Sauce

984 kilojoules/235 calories per serving

300ml (½ pint) skim milk

300ml (½ pint) water

1 tspn cracked black pepper

1 clove garlic, crushed

125g (4oz) polenta

30g (1oz) grated Parmesan cheese

2 tspn oil

1 onion, peeled and chopped

1 clove garlic, crushed, extra

125g (4oz) mushrooms, sliced

¼ tspn ground chilli powder

1 cup tinned tomatoes and their juice

thyme for garnish

1 Place milk, water, pepper and garlic in a small saucepan over moderate heat and bring to the boil. Remove from the heat, cover and stand for 20 minutes. Strain milk into a medium saucepan.

2 Add the polenta and stir over moderate heat, until boiling. Reduce heat and simmer 5 minutes.

3 Pour the polenta onto a greased and lined 20cm (8in) round baking dish or tray, spread out evenly and set aside to cool.

4 Sprinkle polenta with the cheese and bake in a moderate oven for 15 minutes. Cut polenta into wedges and place on serving plate.

5 For the sauce: Heat the oil in a medium frying pan over moderate heat. Add the onion, garlic, mushrooms and chilli, cook for 3 minutes. Add the tomatoes and cook for a further 3 minutes, pour sauce into serving bowl. Garnish with fresh thyme if desired.

Serves 4

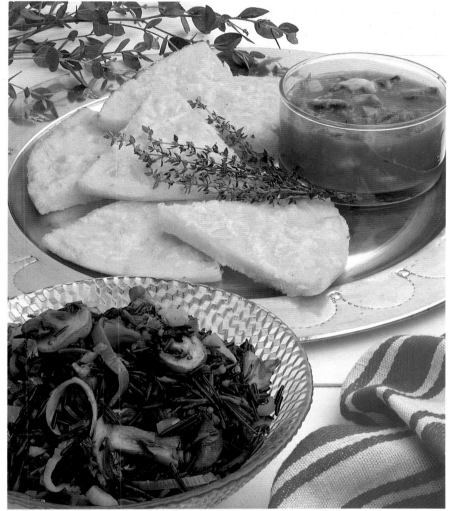

Top: Polenta with Mushroom Sauce. Bottom: Wild Rice and Mushroom Salad

Herbed Zucchini (Courgette) and Lentil Casserole

1005 kilojoules/240 calories per serving

185g (6oz) red lentils

¾ cup chopped onion

1 cup chopped celery

2 tspn safflower oil

125g (4oz) freshly shelled peas

250g (½lb) zucchini (courgette), sliced

1½ tblspn plain flour

3 tblspn chopped fresh parsley

2 tblspn chopped fresh basil

1 tspn chopped fresh thyme (optional)

salt

pepper

freshly squeezed lemon juice (optional)

1 Rinse lentils under cold running water, place in a saucepan with plenty of water to cover. Bring to a boil, reduce heat to a simmer. Cook until lentils are tender, about 30 minutes. Drain, reserve stock.

2 Combine onion, celery and oil in a casserole, saute gently until vegetables are softened, about 5 minutes. Add peas, zucchini and lentils. Add flour, cook 2 minutes, stirring constantly.

3 Stir in 300ml (½ pint) of the reserved lentil stock, followed by parsley, basil and thyme, if used. Cover, cook until vegetables are tender, about 15 minutes. Season to taste with salt and freshly ground pepper, and lemon juice, if used. Serve hot.

Serves 4

VEGETARIAN

Vegetarian dishes tend to be far lower in kilojoules than meat based meals. You'll find these recipes packed full of flavour and satisfying too.

Potatoes Stuffed with Spinach and Cheese

1507 kilojoules/360 calories per serving

4 large potatoes, scrubbed

250g (½lb) spinach, cut into thin strips

1 egg, lightly beaten

200g (6½oz) cottage cheese

30g (1oz) unsalted butter

60g (2oz) mature Cheddar cheese, grated

1 tblspn chopped parsley

1 tblspn chopped chives

salt

pepper

1 Puncture potatoes with a skewer, bake on a rack in a 200°C (400°F) oven until tender, about 1-1½ hours, depending on size.

2 Place spinach in a steamer over boiling water, cover pan securely, steam 3 minutes, drain, squeeze out any excess moisture in a tea-towel.

3 Cut potatoes in half lengthwise. Scoop out flesh, careful not to break skin, reserve skins. Mash flesh, stir in spinach, egg, cottage cheese, butter, Cheddar cheese, parsley and chives. Season to taste with salt and freshly ground pepper.

4 Pile mixture into potato shells, bake in a 180°C (350°F) oven until heated through, about 20 minutes. Serve hot.

Serves 4

Zucchini (Courgette) Crepes with Ricotta Chive Filling

1047 kilojoules/250 calories per serving

2 zucchini (courgette), grated

¼ cup plain flour

3 eggs

¼ cup freshly grated Parmesan cheese

½ cup skim milk

¼ tspn ground nutmeg

1 cup low fat ricotta cheese

1 tblspn freshly squeezed lime juice

2 tblspn chopped chives

¼ tspn cracked black pepper

1 Sprinkle zucchini with 1 tablespoon salt and let stand for 15 minutes. Dry zucchini on paper towels.

2 Place the flour in a large bowl, make a well in the centre, add the eggs, zucchini, cheese, milk and nutmeg, stir ingredients until mixture is smooth.

3 Heat a non-stick frying pan, pour ¼ cup of zucchini mixture into pan to make a large crepe. Cook for 1 minute each side. Repeat with remaining mixture.

4 Beat the ricotta cheese with the lime juice, chives and pepper. Spread 2 tablespoons of the mixture onto each crepe, roll up and serve with a small salad.

Serves 4

Zucchini (Courgette) Crepes with Ricotta Chive Filling

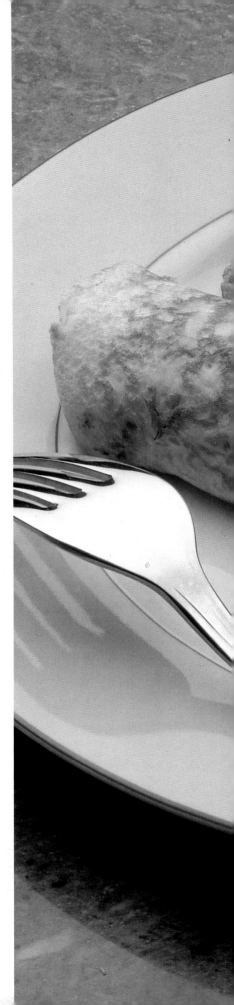

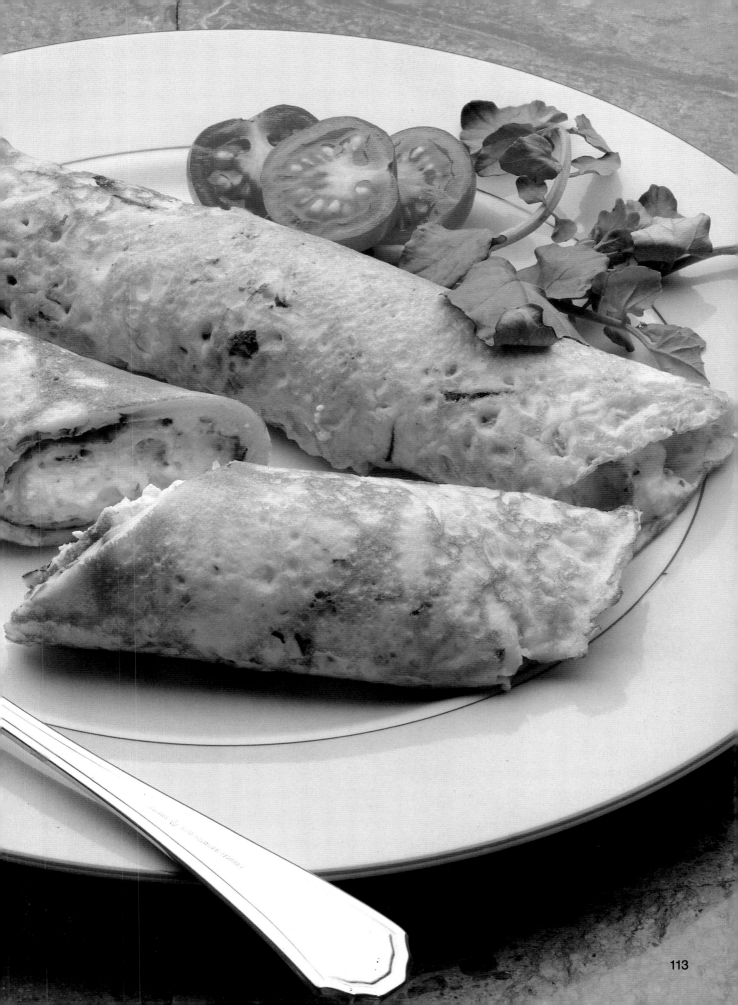

English Vegetable Casserole

670 kilojoules/160 calories per serving

1 tblspn oil

1 onion, peeled and chopped

2 tblspn plain flour

2 cups tinned tomatoes

1 cup tomato puree

1 tblspn chopped fresh thyme

¼ tspn black pepper

1 leek, sliced, white part only

4 spring onions (scallions), chopped

4 carrots, peeled, sliced into thin strips

1 cup button mushrooms, sliced

3 stalks celery, sliced into thin strips

1 Heat the oil in a large frying pan over a moderate heat and cook the onion for 3 minutes. Sprinkle the flour over the onion and cook, stirring constantly for 2 minutes.

2 Add the tomatoes, puree, thyme and pepper, cook for a further 5 minutes.

3 Add the leeks, spring onions, carrots, mushrooms and celery, transfer casserole to an ovenproof dish, cover and cook in a moderate oven for 35 minutes. Garnish with fresh thyme sprigs if desired.

Serves 4

Cauliflower Gratin with Hazelnuts

837 kilojoules/200 calories per serving

1 medium cauliflower, divided into flowerets

1 tspn peanut oil

1 onion, chopped

2 small cloves garlic, finely chopped

60g (2oz) hazelnuts, roughly chopped

60g (2oz) ground hazelnuts

1 tblspn tamari (see note)

1 tspn chopped fresh oregano

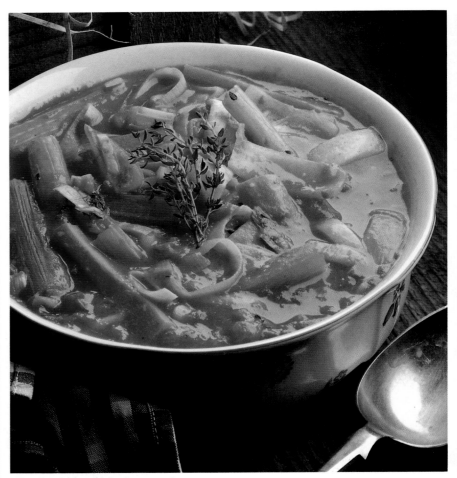

English Vegetable Casserole

1 Boil, steam or microwave cauliflower until just tender, but still crisp. Reserve any cooking liquid. Arrange flowerets into an ovenproof dish.

2 Heat oil in a frying pan, add onion and garlic, saute until golden, about 5 minutes. Add chopped hazelnuts, saute a further 4 minutes. Spoon over the cauliflower.

3 Add enough water to reserved cooking liquid to make up 300ml (½pint). Pour into a processor, add ground hazelnuts, tamari and oregano. Blend, pour over cauliflower.

4 Bake in a 180°C (350°F) oven for 20-25 minutes, or until top is golden. Serve hot.

Note: Tamari is like soy sauce, but stronger in flavour. It is available in health food shops and Asian food stores.

Serves 4

Buckwheat Pancakes with Kumera (Sweet Potato)

1675 kilojoules/400 calories per serving

500g (1lb) kumera (sweet potato)

2 tblspn peanut oil

1 onion, chopped

1 red capsicum (pepper), seeded, chopped

nutmeg

2 tblspn dessicated coconut

PANCAKE BATTER

300ml (½pint) skim milk

1 tspn safflower oil

1 egg

60g (2oz) wholemeal flour

60g (2oz) buckwheat flour

1 Cook kumera in very lightly salted boiling water until tender, about 20 minutes. Drain, reserve ⅓ cup of the cooking liquid. Peel kumera and mash.

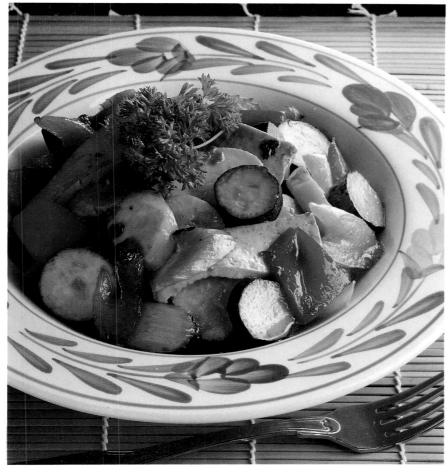

Stir-fry Vegetables with Marinated Tofu

2 Combine oil, onion and capsicum in a large frying pan. Saute until soft, about 5 minutes. Season to taste with nutmeg, cook a further 3 minutes, stirring from time to time.

3 In a large bowl, blend coconut with reserved hot cooking liquid. Add onion and capsicum mixture, stir in mashed kumera. Mix well. Cover bowl, keep warm.

4 To make batter: Combine milk, oil and egg in a processor, blend 30 seconds. Add flours in one batch, process 30 seconds.

5 Lightly grease a 18cm (7in) crepe pan, pour in 2 tablespoons of the batter, cook over medium heat until top has set. Flip over with a spatula, cook other side for 1 minute. Keep warm while cooking remaining pancakes.

6 Put 2 tablespoons of the filling into each pancake, roll up and serve immediately.

Serves 4

Stir-fry Vegetables with Marinated Tofu

1089 kilojoules/260 calories per serving

¼ cup soy sauce

2 tblspn Worcestershire sauce

2 tblspn honey

1 tblspn tomato paste

250g (½lb) firm tofu, cut into slices

4 stalks celery, sliced

2 red capsicum (pepper), seeded, cut into pieces

4 zucchini (courgette), sliced

1 cup baby yellow squash, cut in halves

1 tblspn chopped fresh parsley

1 In a medium bowl, combine the soy sauce, Worcestershire sauce, honey and tomato paste, mix well. Add the tofu, cover, refrigerate and marinate for 2 hours. Remove tofu from marinade and set aside.

2 Pour the marinade into a large frying pan. Heat until the marinade simmers and is reduced by half.

3 Add the celery, capsicum, zucchini and squash, cook for 3 minutes, add the tofu and cook for a further 1 minute. Stir in parsley and serve immediately.

Serves 4

Hungarian Bean Casserole

921 kilojoules/220 calories per serving

185g (6oz) baby lima beans, soaked overnight

1 onion, chopped

1 tblspn olive oil

1 clove garlic, finely chopped

¼ tspn chilli flakes

3 red capsicum (peppers), cut into strips

250g (½lb) button mushrooms, sliced

1 potato, cut into 1cm (½in) cubes

1 tblspn paprika

1½ tblspn tomato puree

salt

pepper

1 Drain beans, cover with plenty of cold water, bring to a boil, reduce heat to a simmer, cover, cook until beans are tender, about 1 hour, depending on age of beans. Drain, reserve cooking liquid.

2 In a large casserole, saute onion in oil until golden, about 5 minutes. Add garlic, chilli flakes, capsicum and mushrooms, saute until softened, about 5 minutes. Cover, cook over a very low heat for 15 minutes.

3 Add beans, potato, paprika and tomato puree, moisten with ½ a cup of the reserved bean liquid. Simmer until potatoes are tender, about 30 minutes, adding more bean liquid if necessary.

4 Season to taste with salt and freshly ground pepper. Serve hot.

Serves 4

Rice and Pimento Terrine

837 kilojoules/200 calories per serving

2 tspn butter

1 onion, chopped

4 cups cooked rice

1 cup skim milk

3 eggs

1 tspn sambal oelek (chilli paste)

¼ cup freshly grated pecorino cheese

2 tblspn chopped fresh parsley

420g (13½ oz) can pimentos, drained

1 Melt the butter in a medium frying pan, add the onions, cook until tender.

2 In a large bowl, combine the rice, milk, eggs, sambal oelek, cheese, parsley and cooked onions, mix well.

3 Grease and line a loaf tin. Pour ⅓ of the rice mixture into the tin. Place ½ the pimentos on top of rice, then top with another ⅓ of the rice mixture. Place the remaining pimentos on top of rice and top with the remaining rice mixture.

4 Bake in a moderate oven for 35-40 minutes. Cook in tin for 10 minutes before turning out. Serve warm or cold.

Serves 8

Spaghetti with Lentil Bolognese

2177 kilojoules/520 calories per serving

185g (6oz) red lentils

1 onion, chopped

2 cloves garlic, crushed

2 tspn olive oil

1 tspn ground turmeric

400g (13oz) can tomatoes, with juice

2 tspn chopped fresh oregano

¼ cup dry red wine

salt

pepper

375g (¾lb) wholemeal spaghetti

30g (1oz) freshly grated Parmesan cheese

1 Place lentils in a saucepan with 1¾ cup water. Bring to a boil, reduce heat to a simmer, cover, cook until lentils have cooked to a puree, about 30 minutes.

2 Saute onion and garlic in oil until onion is golden, about 5 minutes. Add turmeric and lentils, cook a further 5 minutes.

3 Stir in tomatoes, breaking them up with a wooden spoon, then tomato juice, oregano and red wine. Bring to a boil, reduce heat to a simmer, cook 10 minutes. Season to taste with salt and freshly ground pepper.

4 Meanwhile, cook spaghetti in plenty of lightly salted boiling water until al dente, about 12 minutes. Drain, place in a heated bowl, pour over lentil sauce, toss well. Serve hot, sprinkled with Parmesan.

Serves 4

Parsley and Chickpea Patties with Yoghurt Sauce

1151 kilojoules/275 calories per serving

150g (5oz) chickpeas, soaked overnight, drained

2 tblspn parsley, chopped

4 spring onions (scallions), chopped

3 tblspn freshly squeezed lime juice

1 large egg

1 tblspn flour

1 tspn ground cumin

1 tblspn chopped fresh coriander

¾ cup dried breadcrumbs

¼ cup oil

1 cup natural low fat yoghurt

1 clove garlic, crushed

1 tblspn freshly squeezed lemon juice

1 tspn finely chopped chives

1 Place chickpeas in a large saucepan, cover with water and simmer for 1 hour. Drain.

2 Place chickpeas into a food processor, add the parsley, spring onions, lime juice, egg, flour, cumin and coriander, puree until smooth, or until binding.

3 Roll tablespoonfuls of mixture into balls, roll in the breadcrumbs and flatten using the palm of your hand.

4 Heat the oil in a medium frying pan. Add the patties and cook over moderate heat for 3 minutes each side. Drain well on paper towels.

5 To make sauce: Mix together the yoghurt, garlic, lemon juice and chives, pour over patties.

Serves 4

Ragout of Summer Vegetables

377 kilojoules/90 calories per serving

125g (4oz) French beans, topped and tailed

125g (4oz) sugar snap peas, topped and tailed

1 tblspn extra virgin olive oil

1 Spanish onion, thinly sliced

2 cloves garlic, crushed

24 baby onions, peeled

18 baby carrots, peeled

1 sprig tarragon

⅓ cup dry white wine

1 tspn sugar

½ red capsicum (pepper), cut into thin strips

½ yellow capsicum (pepper), cut into thin strips

2 artichoke hearts, drained, quartered

¼ cup coarsely chopped continental parsley

¼ cup coarsely chopped fresh basil

up to ¼ cup freshly squeezed lemon juice

salt

pepper

1 Cook beans in lightly salted boiling water until just tender, but still crisp, about 3 minutes. Remove from pan with a slotted spoon, refresh under cold running water, drain, set aside.

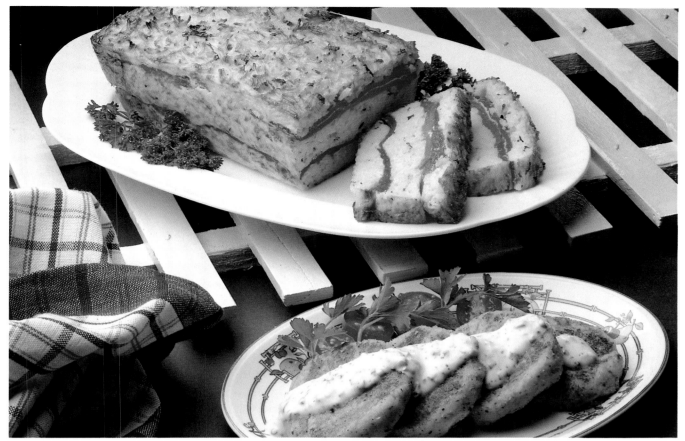

Left: Rice and Pimento Terrine. Right: Parsley and Chickpea Patties with Yoghurt Sauce

2 Cook sugar snap peas in the same water, no longer than 1-2 minutes. Drain, refresh under cold running water. Add peas to beans.

3 In a large casserole combine oil, onion, garlic, baby onions, carrots and the tarragon and thyme sprigs. Cover, cook over very low heat until vegetables are softened, about 5 minutes.

4 Add ¼ cup of the wine and the sugar, mix in well. Cover, cook until vegetables are just tender, stirring from time to time, about 20 minutes.

5 Stir in red and yellow capsicum, cover, cook until softened, about 5 minutes. Add artichokes, reserved beans and peas and remaining tablespoon wine. Cook just long enough to heat through.

6 Remove from the heat, stir in parsley and basil, season to taste with lemon juice, salt and freshly ground pepper. Serve hot or at room temperature.

Serves 6

Pumpkin Gratin

1507 kilojoules/360 calories per serving
1.5kg (3lb) butternut pumpkin
salt
pepper
1 tspn olive oil
1 cup chopped onion
6 tblspn dry white wine
6 tblspn degreased chicken stock
1 cup milk
8 thin slices of a baguette, toasted
125g (4oz) grated mature Cheddar cheese
1 tblspn freshly grated Parmesan cheese
dill for garnish

1 Halve pumpkin lengthwise, remove seeds. Place pumpkin in an oven dish, cut side up. Season to taste with salt and freshly ground pepper, cover securely with foil. Bake in a 200°C (400°F) oven until flesh is easily pierced, about 1 hour. Cool slightly.

2 Meanwhile, combine oil, onion and half a teaspoon water in a saucepan. Cover, cook over medium heat until onion is softened, about 5 minutes.

3 Add wine, bring to a boil, cook uncovered until liquid is reduced by half. Off the heat, add stock and milk, season to taste with salt and freshly ground pepper. Bring to a boil, keep simmering.

4 Remove chunks of flesh from half the pumpkin with a big spoon, place in a casserole. Pour over half the onion and milk mixture, arrange 4 pieces of toast on top, sprinkle with half the cheese. Repeat this process with remaining pumpkin, onion and milk mixture, toast and cheese. Sprinkle top with Parmesan.

5 Bake in a 200°C (400°F) oven until top is bubbly and brown. Sprinkle with dill, serve hot.

Serves 4

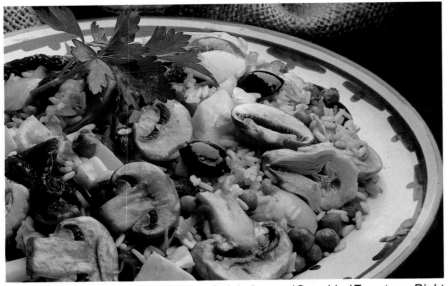

Above: Warm Rice Salad with Peas, Artichokes and Sun-dried Tomatoes. Right Top: Vegetable Terrine. Right Bottom: Eggplant (Aubergine) and Butter Bean Risotto

Eggplant (Aubergine) and Butter Bean Risotto

1256 kilojoules/300 calories per serving

1 tblspn oil

1 tspn poppy seeds

1 tspn mustard seeds

1 cup long grain rice

¼ tspn chilli powder

1 tspn turmeric

1 tspn cumin

1 tspn ground coriander

1 eggplant (aubergine), cut into ½cm (¼in) cubes

½ red capsicum (pepper), seeded and chopped

310g (10oz) can butter beans, rinsed and drained

1½ cups tomato puree

1½ cups degreased chicken stock

½ cup coconut milk

1 tblspn fresh chopped coriander

1 Heat the oil in a large frying pan, add the poppy and mustard seeds and cook until they begin to pop. Add the rice and continue cooking for 5 minutes.

2 In a separate bowl, mix together the chilli powder, turmeric, cumin and coriander with 2 tablespoons of cold water to make a paste. Pour paste over the rice, add eggplant, capsicum and butter beans, mix well and cook for a further 5 minutes.

3 Add 1 cup of water to the tomato puree, stock and coconut milk, add to the pan, cover and simmer for 30-40 minutes, or until rice is cooked and most of the liquid is absorbed. Stir in fresh coriander, serve warm.

Serves 4-6

Vegetable Terrine

607 kilojoules/145 calories per serving

8 large spinach leaves, washed

2 tblspn oil

1½ tblspn plain flour

1¼ cups skim milk

¼ tspn ground nutmeg

¼ tspn black pepper

¼ cup natural low fat yoghurt

2 eggs, lightly beaten

125g (4oz) peas, lightly steamed

125g (4oz) carrots, chopped and cooked

1 Pour boiling water over spinach, drain after 1 minute.

2 Gently heat the oil in a saucepan. Stir in the flour, cook for 30 seconds. Gradually add the milk and bring to the boil, stirring constantly. Season with the nutmeg and pepper.

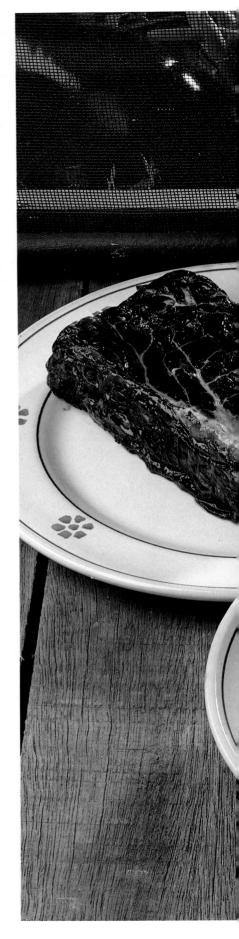

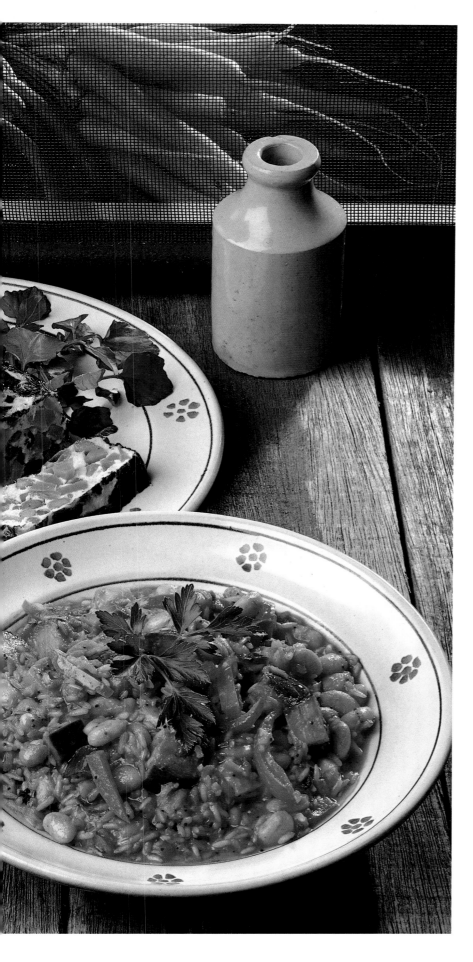

3 Cool slightly, then whisk in the yoghurt and eggs. Add the peas and carrots to the yoghurt sauce.

4 Line a loaf tin with the spinach leaves, reserving one for the top. Pour in the sauce and top with reserved spinach leaf. Fold over the leaves to cover the mixture completely.

5 Place the tin in a bain-marie or a roasting tin filled with about 2.5cm (1in) hot water. Bake for 1 hour. Cool completely before turning out onto a serving plate. Serve cold.

Makes 8 slices

Warm Rice Salad with Peas, Artichokes and Sun-dried Tomatoes

1319 kilojoules/315 calories per serving

1 tblspn olive oil

3 tblspn white wine vinegar

2 tblspn freshly squeezed orange juice

2 cloves garlic, crushed

2 stalks celery, chopped

¼ cup drained and sliced sun-dried tomatoes

½ cup sliced button mushrooms

½ cup quartered yellow squash

½ cup thawed frozen peas

½ cup pawpaw (papaya), cut into 1cm (½in) cubes

1 cup artichokes, drained and cut in halves

2 cups cooked long grain rice

2 large carrots, grated

8 black olives, pitted and sliced

1 Heat the olive oil in a large frying pan, over moderate heat, add the vinegar, orange juice and garlic, cook 1 minute.

2 Add the celery, sun-dried tomatoes, mushrooms, squash and peas, cook for 3 minutes.

3 Add the pawpaw, artichokes and rice, toss well. Stir in the carrot and olives and spoon onto a serving plate. Garnish with a sprig of continental parsley.

Serves 4

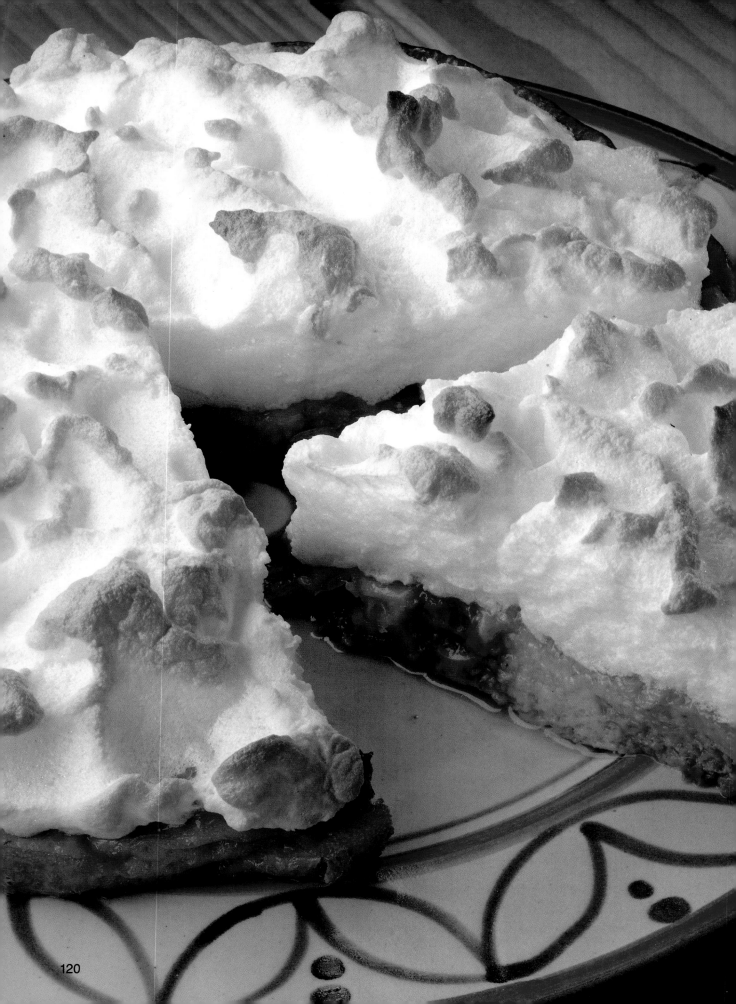

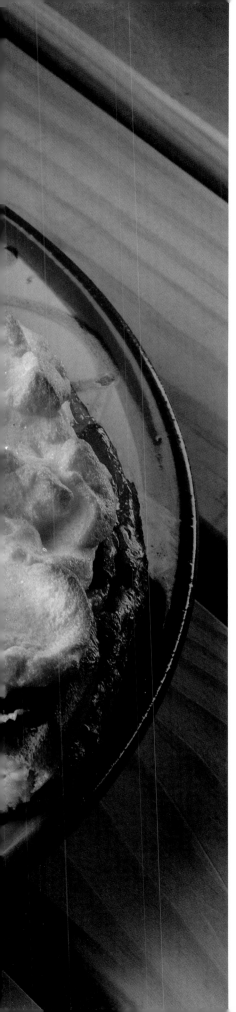

DESSERTS

Just because you're watching your weight doesn't mean you can't enjoy desserts. Try these delightful recipes, they're delicious and won't hurt your waistline.

Amaretto Fruit Frittata with Meringue Topping

502 kilojoules/120 calories per serving

4 eggs

1 tspn castor sugar

3 tblspn Amaretto liqueur

3 tblspn skim milk

¼ cup strawberries, hulled and cut into quarters

¼ cup fresh raspberries

1 orange, peeled and segmented

3 egg-whites

1 Whisk the eggs with the sugar, Amaretto and milk until well combined and sugar has dissolved.

2 Add the strawberries, raspberries and orange segments and pour mixture into a greased 20cm (8in) ovenproof flan dish. Bake in a moderate oven for 20 minutes.

3 Beat egg-whites with an electric mixer until soft peaks form. Spread meringue over the top of frittata and return to oven for 5-7 minutes or until meringue is golden.

Serves 6

Almond Honey Ice-Cream

649 kilojoules/155 calories per serving

3 tblspn honey

2 drops vanilla essence

6 egg yolks

2 cups low-fat skim milk

3 tblspn slivered almonds, toasted and chopped

1 Combine honey, vanilla and egg yolks in a bowl, beat until smooth.

2 Bring milk to a near-boil in the top of a double boiler. Remove ¼ cup of the hot milk, stir into the egg yolk mixture.

3 Stir egg yolk mixture into the milk in one batch, stir over simmering water for 3-5 minutes, until custard coats the back of a spoon. Remove from heat, allow to cool. Stir in almonds.

4 Pour custard into an ice-cream machine, freeze according to manufacturer's instructions. Spoon into a container, cover tightly, place in freezer. When serving, allow to soften slightly in refrigerator for 20 minutes.

Serves 6

Amaretto Fruit Frittata with Meringue Topping

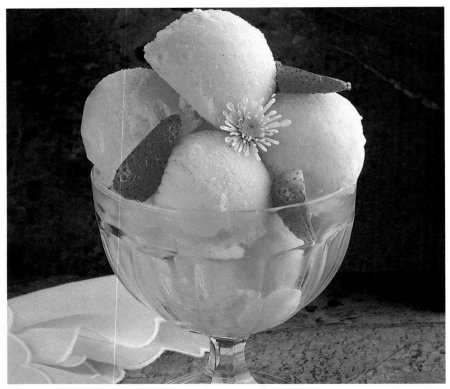

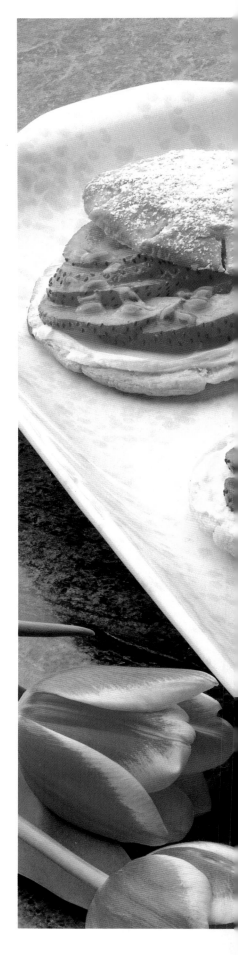

Above: Honey Vanilla Ice-Cream. Right: Cream Cheese Strawberry Tartlets

Honey Vanilla Ice-Cream

963 kilojoules/230 calories per serving

5 egg yolks

2 tblspn honey

1 tspn vanilla essence

2 cups low fat skim milk

8 strawberries, halved

1 Mix the egg yolks with the honey and vanilla in the top of a double saucepan. Add the milk and whisk for about 8 minutes over simmering water until mixture thickens slightly.

2 Pour mixture into ice-cream maker and freeze according to instructions.

3 If no ice-cream maker is availabe, freeze mixture for 1 hour, remove from freezer, beat mixture with electric mixer, return to freezer. Repeat this process every hour for three hours. Freeze until ready to serve.

4 Garnish with strawberries if desired.

Serves 4

Cream Cheese Strawberry Tartlets

879 kilojoules/210 calories per serving

1 sheet frozen short crust pastry, thawed

50g (1¾ oz) lite cream cheese

100g (3½oz) ricotta cheese

1 tblspn castor sugar

2 tspn vanilla essence

1 cup strawberries, hulled and sliced

1 passionfruit

1 Using an 8-10cm (¾in) diameter cutter (or a glass can be used), cut out 4 rounds of pastry from pastry sheet. Decorate pastry edge by pinching and bake on greased oven tray for 10 minutes in a moderately hot oven. Leave pastry rounds on a rack to cool.

2 Meanwhile, beat the cream cheese, ricotta cheese, sugar and vanilla essence together until smooth.

3 Spread the top of each pastry round with the cheese mixture and top with strawberry slices and passionfruit.

Makes 4

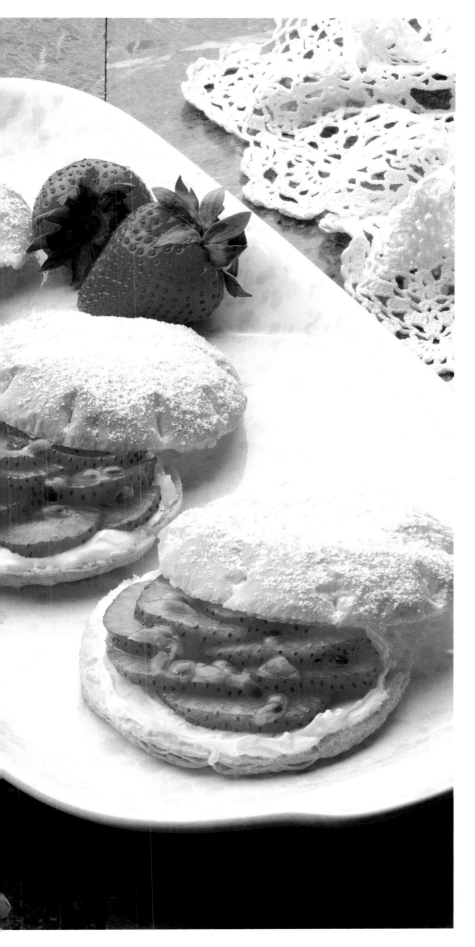

Rockmelon (Cantaloupe) Sorbet with Blueberry Sauce

607 kilojoules/145 calories per serving

SORBET

1.5kg (3lb) rockmelon (cantaloupe), peeled, seeded, roughly cut up

¾ cup sugar

salt

1 tblspn freshly squeezed lemon juice

SAUCE

3 cups fresh blueberries

1 tblspn freshly squeezed lemon juice

⅓ cup port

1 To make the sorbet: Puree rockmelon in a food processor until smooth, scraping down sides once.

2 Place 1 cup of the puree in a saucepan, add sugar and a pinch of salt. Cook over medium heat until sugar has dissolved, stirring continuously.

3 Pour into a large bowl, blend with remaining puree. Cover bowl, refrigerate until chilled. Stir in lemon juice. Transfer to an ice-cream machine, freeze according to manufacturer's instructions.

4 To make the sauce: Combine 2 cups of the blueberries in a saucepan with the lemon juice and port. Bring to a simmer, cook until blueberries are tender, about 5 minutes.

5 Remove half the blueberries from the pan, strain back into the pan through a sieve. Discard pulp.

6 Stir uncooked berries into the pan, heat through gently. Serve warm with sorbet.

Serves 8

Orange Rice Cream

795 kilojoules/ 190 calories per serving

150g (5oz) short grain white rice

600ml (1 pint) skim milk

1 tblspn finely grated orange rind

1 cup freshly squeezed orange juice

2 tspn honey

¼ tspn ground cinnamon

½ cup skim milk, extra

8 strawberries for garnish

1 Place the rice, milk, orange rind, orange juice, honey and cinnamon in a large saucepan. Bring mixture to the boil over moderate heat, stirring constantly. Reduce heat, cover and simmer for 40 minutes or until rice is cooked and the liquid is absorbed.

2 Stir in the extra milk and cook until almost absorbed. Spoon into serving glasses and garnish with sliced strawberries.

Serves 4

Grand Marnier Souffle

1172 kilojoules/280 calories per serving

45g (1½oz) butter

1 tblspn grated orange rind

¼ cup castor sugar

3 tspn cornflour

1½ tblspn plain flour

1 tblspn freshly squeezed orange juice

3 tblspn Grand Marnier

¾ cup skim milk

3 eggs, separated

3 tspn gelatine, dissolved in 2 tblspn warm water

1 Beat butter with rind and sugar in a small bowl until light and fluffy. Beat in the flour, orange juice and Grand Marnier.

2 Heat the milk in a medium saucepan over moderate heat. Stir in spoonfuls of the butter mixture until mixture boils and thickens. Cool mixture slightly, whisk in egg yolks and dissolved gelatine.

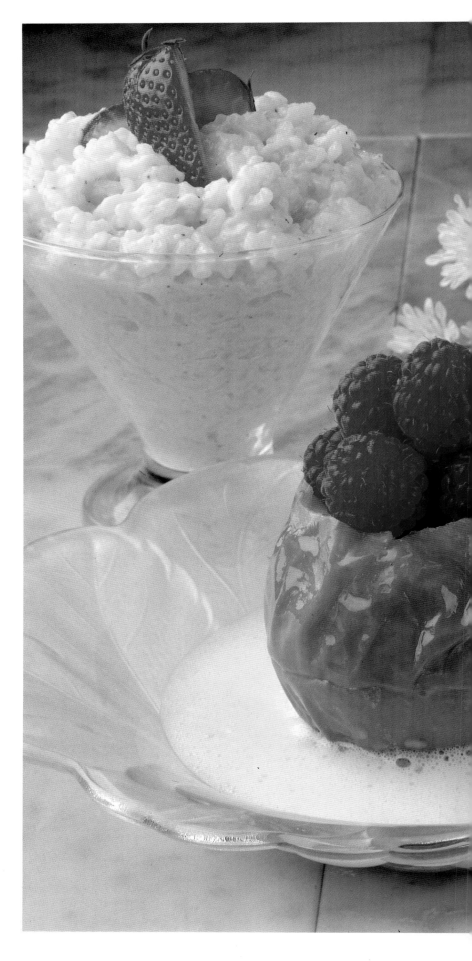

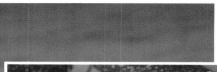

Left Top: Orange Rice Cream. Left Bottom: Foamy Baked Apples with Sultanas. Below: Grand Marnier Souffle

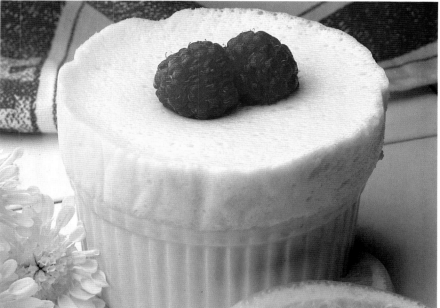

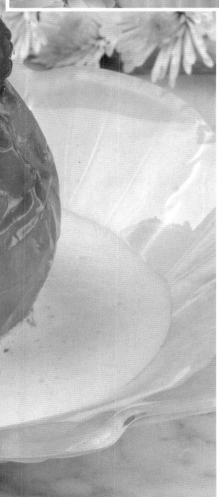

3 Beat the egg-whites in a large bowl until soft peaks form. Fold egg-whites into custard mixture.

4 Grease 4 ½-cup capacity souffle dishes and tie a band of grease-proof paper around the top of the dishes, to stand 5cm (2in) above the rim.

5 Pour mixture into dishes, chill until set. Remove paper carefully and garnish with fresh raspberries.

Serves 4

Coffee Zabaglione

398 kilojoules/95 calories per serving

3 eggs

⅓ cup espresso coffee, cooled

¼ cup Marsala

1 tblspn sugar

1 Separate eggs. Combine egg yolks, coffee and Marsala in a bowl, beat until smooth.

2 Beat egg-whites with the sugar until stiff peaks form, fold into egg yolk mixture.

3 Pour into 4 shallow champagne glasses, serve immediately.

Serves 4

Foamy Baked Apples with Sultanas

523 kilojoules/125 calories per serving

4 large green apples

4 tblspn sultanas

1 large egg

½ cup freshly squeezed orange juice

1 orange for garnish

¼ cup fresh raspberries for garnish

1 Wash and core apples using a knife. Make an incision in the apple skin, cut right around the centre.

2 Place the apples in a baking dish, fill the centre cavity with sultanas and bake in a moderate oven for about 25 minutes.

3 Meanwhile, place the egg and orange juice in the top of a double saucepan and whisk until mixture is slightly thickened and foamy.

4 Serve sauce over apples and garnish with orange slices and fresh raspberries.

Serves 4

Flambe Strawberries

377 kilojoules/90 calories per serving

1 tblspn unsalted butter

1 tblspn honey

2 tspn Cointreau

½ tspn grated orange rind

2 tspn water

1½ cups strawberries, halved

2 tspn warmed brandy

1 In a frying pan, combine butter, honey, Cointreau, orange rind and water. Bring to a boil, add strawberries.

2 Saute for 1 minute, sprinkle with brandy, light with a match. Baste strawberries with liquid until flame dies down.

3 Spoon into dessert dishes, serve immediately.

Serves 4

Apple Crumble with Oat Topping

544 kilojoules/130 calories per serving

1/4 cup rolled oats, roughly chopped

1/3 cup dark brown sugar

1 tblspn plain flour

salt

1 tblspn unsalted butter, melted

625g (1lb 4oz) Granny Smith apples

1/2 tspn cinnamon

nutmeg

1 In a small bowl, combine oats, 2 tablespoons of the sugar, flour, a pinch of salt and the butter. Mix well, set aside.

2 Peel and core apples, cut into 1cm (1/2in) thick slices. Mix in remaining 2 tablespoons sugar, cinnamon and nutmeg.

3 Place apples in a flan dish, sprinkle topping over. Bake in a 230°C (450°F) oven until top is crisp and brown, about 20 minutes. Serve hot.

Serves 6

Prune Souffle

481 kilojoules/115 calories per serving

2 tspn unsalted butter, melted

2 tblspn castor sugar

250g (1/2lb) pitted prunes

1/4 cup Armagnac or brandy

10cm (4in) strip orange zest

3 egg-whites, at room temperature

salt

2 tblspn castor sugar, extra

icing sugar for dusting

1 Brush an 8-cup capacity souffle dish with melted butter, sprinkle with sugar, rotate dish in your hands to spread sugar evenly. Set aside.

2 Combine prunes, Armagnac and orange zest in a saucepan with 1/2 cup water. Slowly bring to a simmer. Cover, remove from the heat. Allow to stand for 20 minutes.

3 Discard orange zest, blend prunes and liquid in a processor to a lumpy consistency.

4 Beat egg-whites with a pinch of salt until soft peaks form. Add 1 tablespoon sugar, beat until well incorporated, add remaining tablespoon sugar. Beat until stiff peaks form.

5 Fold 1/2 cup of the whites into prunes to lighten puree. Fold prune mixture lightly but thoroughly into remaining egg-whites. Run your thumb along top inside to push mixture away from rim. This will enable the souffle to rise more easily.

6 Bake in a 200°C (400°F) oven on a low rack until golden and well risen, about 15 minutes. Dust lightly with icing sugar. Serve immediately.

Serves 6

Fresh Orange with Grand Marnier Snow

523 kilojoules/125 calories per serving

3 large oranges

4 egg-whites

1/2 cup icing sugar

1/4 cup Grand Marnier

1 tblspn freshly squeezed lemon juice

1 Grate the zest of one of the oranges, set aside. Peel all the oranges, remove all pith and membranes. Work over a bowl to catch juices. Divide segments among 6 shallow champagne glasses, cover, refrigerate.

2 Beat egg-whites with a hand-held electric beater until soft peaks form. Add sugar gradually, continue beating until all sugar has been incorporated. Beat until stiff, then beat in Grand Marnier and lemon juice.

3 Place generous dollops of the snow on top of oranges, sprinkle with zest. Serve immediately.

Serves 6

Berry Yoghurt

209 kilojoules/50 calories per serving

1 egg-white

1 tblspn castor sugar

1 cup mixed fresh berries

1/2 cup plain low fat yoghurt

1 Beat the egg-white with the sugar until light and fluffy.

2 Add the berries and beat until mixture is smooth, about 1 minute.

3 Fold in the yoghurt and spoon into chilled serving glasses. Serve immediately.

Serves 4

Poached Fruit Compote

712 kilojoules/170 calories per serving

2 cups fruity white wine

3/4 cup green grapes

3/4 cup drained, canned peach slices

3/4 cup strawberries, hulled and halved

1 tblspn sugar

1 tblspn butter, cut into pieces

1 tblspn orange rind, thinly sliced

1 Heat the wine in a medium saucepan over moderate heat until simmering.

2 Add the grapes, peach slices and strawberries and simmer for 30 seconds. Transfer fruit with a slotted spoon to a bowl and cover.

3 Add sugar to the liquid, boil over high heat until syrupy, about 7 minutes.

4 Swirl in butter pieces and orange rind and pour over the fruit. Serve immediately.

Serves 4

Top: Berry Yoghurt.
Bottom: Poached Fruit Compote

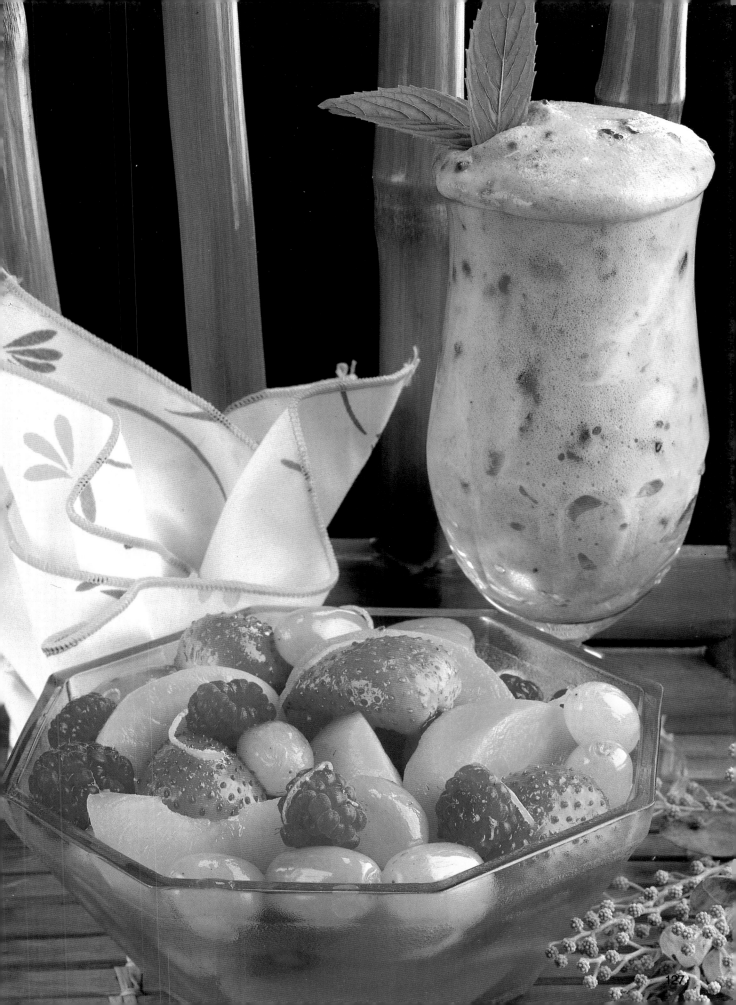

TEMPERATURE AND MEASUREMENT EQUIVALENTS

OVEN TEMPERATURES

	Fahrenheit	Celsius
Very slow	250°	120°
Slow	275–300°	140–150°
Moderately slow	325°	160°
Moderate	350°	180°
Moderately hot	375°	190°
Hot	400–450°	200–230°
Very hot	475–500°	250–260°

CUP AND SPOON MEASURES

Measures given in our recipes refer to the standard metric cup and spoon sets approved by the Standards Association of Australia.

A basic metric cup set consists of 1 cup, ½ cup, ⅓ cup and ¼ cup sizes.

The basic spoon set comprises 1 tablespoon, 1 teaspoon, ½ teaspoon and ¼ teaspoon. These sets are available at leading department, kitchen and hardware stores.

IMPERIAL/METRIC CONVERSION CHART

MASS (WEIGHT)

(Approximate conversions for cookery purposes.)

Imperial	Metric	Imperial	Metric
½ oz	15 g	10 oz	315 g
1 oz	30 g	11 oz	345 g
2 oz	60 g	12 oz (¾ lb)	375 g
3 oz	90 g	13 oz	410 g
4 oz (¼ lb)	125 g	14 oz	440 g
5 oz	155 g	15 oz	470 g
6 oz	185 g	16 oz (1 lb)	500 g (0.5 kg)
7 oz	220 g	24 oz (1½ lb)	750 g
8 oz (½ lb)	250 g	32 oz (2 lb)	1000 g (1 kg)
9 oz	280 g	3 lb	1500 g (1.5 kg)

METRIC CUP AND SPOON SIZES

Cup	Spoon
¼ cup = 60 ml	¼ teaspoon = 1.25 ml
⅓ cup = 80 ml	½ teaspoon = 2.5 ml
½ cup = 125 ml	1 teaspoon = 5 ml
1 cup = 250 ml	1 tablespoon = 20 ml

LIQUIDS

Imperial	Cup*	Metric
1 fl oz		30 ml
2 fl oz	¼ cup	60 ml
3 fl oz		100 ml
4 fl oz	½ cup	125 ml

LIQUIDS (cont'd)

Imperial	Cup*	Metric
5 fl oz (¼ pint)		150 ml
6 fl oz	¾ cup	200 ml
8 fl oz	1 cup	250 ml
10 fl oz (½ pint)	1¼ cups	300 ml
12 fl oz	1½ cups	375 ml
14 fl oz	1¾ cups	425 ml
15 fl oz		475 ml
16 fl oz	2 cups	500 ml
20 fl oz (1 pint)	2½ cups	600 ml

* Cup measures are the same in Imperial and Metric.

LENGTH

Inches	Centimetres	Inches	Centimetres
¼	0.5	7	18
½	1	8	20
¾	2	9	23
1	2.5	10	25
1½	4	12	30
2	5	14	35
2½	6	16	40
3	8	18	45
4	10	20	50
6	15		

NB: 1 cm = 10 mm.